T0110730

NEUROPHILOSOPHY OF CONSCIOUSNESS, VOL. V AND YOGI

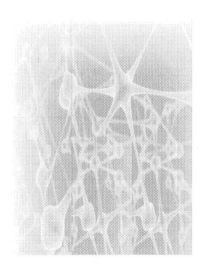

Dr. Angell O. de la Sierra, Esq.

Order this book online at www.trafford.com
or email orders@trafford.com

Most Trafford titles are also available at major online book retailers.

© Copyright 2013 Dr. Angell O. de la Sierra, Esq.
All rights reserved. No part of this publication may be reproduced, stored in a retrieval
system, or transmitted, in any form or by any means, electronic, mechanical, photocopying,
recording, or otherwise, without the written prior permission of the author.

Printed in the United States of America.

ISBN: 978-1-4669-7857-7 (sc)
ISBN: 978-1-4669-7856-0 (e)

Trafford rev. 02/01/2013

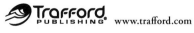

www.trafford.com

North America & international
toll-free: 1 888 232 4444 (USA & Canada)
phone: 250 383 6864 ♦ fax: 812 355 4082

CONTENTS

PROLOGUE

In this continuation of our speculations and conjectures about brain dynamics as it pertains the attainment of the introspective self conscious state and the concomitant brain proto language faculty activation—both 'sine qua non' antecedents to the decision making process—we are now trying to get a clearer picture about what seems to our species confusion of consciously experiencing two simultaneous but opposing perspectives of the same existential 4-d reality and how it may impact the conscious free judgment on the priority to be assigned to any important and relevant issue to the human species. Which one should we adopt to guide our lives today and the 'day after tomorrow'? Of course we are more concerned with the above average responsible citizen looking beyond the conveniences of a quotidian hedonistic Sartrean existentialism where pleasurable enjoyment is routinely satisfied ahead of known but ignored necessities for the lasting survival of the human species generations ahead. How can we reconcile these seemingly opposing views we need to take into account? This realistic approach is called compromise, hybridization or complementarity and the assumption that hidden variables—if any—beyond human brain phenomenological or combinatorial threshold would always bring Heisenberg-type uncertainties to reckon with. These can be either the choice of exclusive biopsychosocial (BPS) imperatives for any living species survival as opposed to the altruistic, spiritual life against self interests of the historical prophets or the more familiar Einstein, Podolsky, Rosen (EPR) complementarities between the **position** of a particulate object of mass (m) and its **momentum** when we try to measure them. Likewise for **energy** and **time.** Underlying these seemingly opposite/contrasting appearances are subthreshold physical interactions. These considerations force you to adopt a quantum statistical probabilistic view of reality relying on falsifiability, predictability and mathematical logic manipulations of symbolic representations of measurable/observed facts. But when it comes to human judgments these coexisting complementarities, i.e., the **subconscious** species survival BPS imperative drives we share with other evolved species to stay alive 'now and then' and the **conscious** species survival across generations sacrifices a few were willing to endure against self interest, resist being framed into coherent rules of metaphysical logic for analysis.

At best, for the ordinary 'Joe Blow' who financially enslave himself to get a college education and maybe a job, the receding 'ultimate truth' seems like the kind of reality which must transcend any familiar mode of thought processing and speech communication, one that unmistakenly must be the result of faultless cognitive processes reserved for the exalted few and literati beings. In our opinion this has been the result of an extremist radicalization of self serving intellectual ideologies, the ideal rationalist world abstraction of an universal reality on the one hand and real 4-d space time existential reality confronting Joe Blow day in and day out with no guarantee that there will be a tomorrow for the surviving, if any. In this volume we continue with our systematic analysis of these complex issues to reinforce our premise that the best possible solution comes from a reconciliation of the extreme views at all levels of organization and the acceptance of what seems to us the natural priorities, a mesoscopic space time reality with serious-minded humans beings at the controls steering the peaceful compliance with human biopsychosocial equilibrium strategies guaranteeing our species survival today and 'the day after tomorrow'. We ask questions like "What exactly do we mean by the 'existence' of an object or event? Do we mean its **physical** identification and phenomenological description in real space time now and/or always? Or is it enough to rely on its probable **metaphysical** logic structure/function explanation when below the threshold of sensory resolution?" Stay tuned . . .

CHAPTER 1

Epistemontological Paradox in Free Choices

What Reality is True?

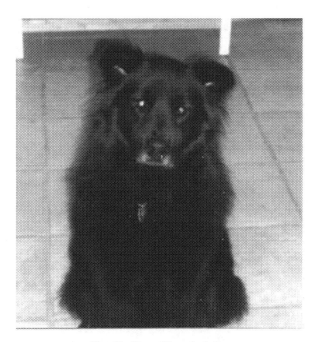

Charlie Boy 'Speaks' Out

INTRODUCTION

What exactly do we mean by the 'existence' of an object or event? Do we mean its **physical** identification and phenomenological description in real space time now and/or always? Or is it enough to rely on its probable **metaphysical** logic structure/function explanation when below the threshold of sensory resolution? Considering the relatively poor sensory resolution our human species brain is endowed with (as compared to other species), would you always rely on the truth value of the complex phenomenological **description** of any object/event? Or would you rather prefer the metaphysical logic **explanation** of the probable structure/function of any complex object/event as conditioned by the relevant circumstances surrounding the human observer and/or the observed/measured? If not yet satisfied, what if both approaches are hybridized as one epistemontological unit where the ontological moiety will only accept falsifiable observations or measurements by normal persons and the epistemological moiety is based on the appropriate mathematical logic deductive conclusions? Or would you rather settle for the inclusion of intuitionistic mathematics logic, possibilities and inductive logic approaches? This is the equivalent of asking if only the immanent quotidian experience is relevant in existential reality, or only the transcendental abstract speculations about a possible future is important or perhaps whether we should be existential realists and accept a compromise focused on the exigent circumstances and requirements of quotidian existential reality? To follow is a brief analysis of the seemingly paradoxical act of conscious free choices.

ARGUMENTATION

What level of cognitive awareness of reality is necessary and convenient to realize one's role as a spouse, parent, neighbor, citizen, etc.? Charlie, my dog, does a wonderful job of our household security surveillance and has earned its living necessities of health, food, shelter, protection and conveniences of perks, toys, trips and love. How many of us would rather freely choose that seemingly 'unchanging' level of Sartrean existence because required adaptive changes are perceived as beyond our control? Nothing wrong if consciously and freely so willed. However, because of the self evident course of evolutionary changes, the Sartrean formula wouldn't work beyond a few generations in obvious detriment to the species survival, unless we yield, like Charlie subconsciously did, and submit to the benevolent enslavement of your freedom. It became then the duty or choice for some historical few to prepare and plan for future changes sacrificing the ongoing 'modern' conveniences of having adopted a democratic, constitutional form of government with all the guarantees of freedom, healthy lives, psychic happiness and social cooperation (bps). This allows for the flourishing of all kinds of institutions and technologies whose aim is to maximize a bps equilibrium and keep all rules of law and analysis clearly spelled out inside a 'safety box' of standards that guide the ongoing generation. But generations evolve and the rules of law and the standards of social guidance need to keep pace with those changes. We need to, under the guidance of the immanent protocol inside the 'safety box', start thinking outside the box in the generation of transcendental rules of species survival today and the day after tomorrow.

The retired senior citizen may erroneously feel that, why change anything, 'what has worked for my generation should be good enough for my grandchildren'. We have all witnessed the role information technology has played in fueling a psychosocial revolution in the non-western world. The new leaders have forged a new standard of biopsychosocial idealism based on metaphysical logic models a supercomputer can simulate. This conceptualization of the ideal leader of tomorrow is the brain child of the physical materialistic faith, mostly mathematicians and theoretical physicists. For them **all** of physical reality, the seen and the unseen, can be reduced to symbolic or sentential logic representations for computers to combine, permute, parse and bingo, there is the new probable survival map or kit for posterity to follow! Life under the new postmodern physical materialist cult will substitute the old dictatorial enslavement deeply rooted on inherited power and riches for the intellectual elites that fuels the monopolistic capitalism ambitions of exploitation of the underground few controlling all means of production. For the new intellectual underground combo—protected by the elected 'politicians for sale'—adopting new and convoluted symbolic abstractions just adds new computer tools of analysis. Unfortunately, the premise of a robotic 'living computer' controlling the human decision making process is delusional if we bother to pay more attention to the real nature of the human species at random and not at the mostly self indulging prophets in the intelligentsia of think tanks of the few 'Mega/Giga societies'. Actually, as it turns out, thinking outside the established physico-mathematical box standards and incorporating the real space time emotional human being existing in quotidian, ongoing reality as part of the standard model equation—as some try in developing and constructing an intuitionistivistic mathematical logic—requires abandoning the comfort of reviewing the familiar and adding another dimension of intellectual activity because it requires getting rid of the crutches supporting our standard views. The 'bps' approach demands practically modifying just about every aspect of our theoretical foundations, from methodology, theorems to technical vocabulary. Are the scholarly professional scientists, academicians and philosophers ready for the constructivism difficulties anticipated with its stricter notion of proof? One needs not deny the value and strength of the 'standard proofs', on the contrary you need to point them out and prove that you can provide a more credible functional solution by partially ignoring the standard proof as specifically relevant. One common point of disagreement is the mathematician's insistence on not having to be concerned as to whether an 'existing *mathematical* object/event' has a physical reality or not, regardless of it being beyond instrumental sensory threshold to describe or not. I submit that it is possible to find algorithms compatible with both the alleged universal classical standards and the realistic intuitionistic approach suggested by our 'bps' brain dynamics model. It should not be surprising to witness the occasional low brow street brawl enacted by fundamentalist religionists of the theosophist and physical materialistic indoctrination/persuasion when they 'analyze' the mathematics of the Axiom of Choice (AC) principle.

Needless to remind the readers that in a cosmology controlled and ruled by a mathematical logic, there is no reality or 'intelligent design' other than that phenomenologically measured or the result of a metaphysical logic parsing among symbolic/sentential logic representations. This leaves no room to accommodate relevant, falsifiable and complex subjective experiences that resist being symbolically framed for deductive mathematical analysis, i.e., anything beyond this 'objective' threshold is a 'mathematical object' with no conceivable physical reality where its phenomenological subjective manifestations just 'emerge'. This is the equivalent of the radical theosophy and their subjective convictions by faith alone that violate all of natural laws, e.g., particulate matter can emerge into 'existence' from a 'vacuum' or we can gain information from an ever-receding linear infinity. Nature abhors both the vacuum and infinities just like it does when conveniently ignoring the physical presence and relevance of the complex human brain in the decision making process. This does not mean that the 'standard' positions are as probably good as they will ever get to be even when we make allowances for our intrinsic brain dynamics sensory and cognitive limitations. But, there is no good reason to stop searching for answers to refine on either of these extremes cosmologies or propose a new one. Is it not obvious that the truth worth of a mathematical statement can only be conceived via a physical brain constructive effort that proves it to be true or not? What else, besides the phenomenologically experienced seems to say my dog Charlie Boy with his own psychosis of curiosity as he inquisitively stares deep into our also curious eyes.

To elaborate further on the example, consider the standard abstract contrivance/notion of an **absolute** non-empty set containing a collection of **all** non-empty sets which 'logically' cannot contain itself. Since our human species cannot yet prove or disprove the existence of open ended infinities or absolute vacuums, we can consciously and intuitively choose to ignore the classical proof and invoke the convenient abstract concept of a transfinity (a perfectly logical probability space time coordinates between infinity and finiteness in spite of the lack of verifiable space time coordinates), so long as it is consistent with mathematical logic and allows for phenomenological predictions of corroborated behavioral experiences or measurements. Iff necessary or convenient one may even choose to assume that there 'exists' a common denominator to all sets to suit my intended other conclusions, crazy things like, if nothing better, all subset members of the set have minimum and maximum dimensional values! Comparing any two invisible physical particles r, s either:

$$r < s \text{ or } r = s \text{ or } r > s.$$

Likewise for any three particles r, u, v either:

$$\text{if } u < v, \text{ then } r > u \text{ or } r < v$$

After all, in our human 4-d mesoscopic real space time world any application ultimately must rely on only finitely many measurements or falsifiable experiences. This is what always happens in applied real time mathematics. What must be remembered is that there is a commitment of the intuitionist mathematician to **construct** not for self indulgence but should always imply a search for the honest probability to **find** the physical reality embedding the abstract intuition.

As a closing argument in this brief non-technical exposition we'd like to dwell on the mathematic purist's classic insistence on the absolute truth value of their proof of the *Law of the Excluded Middle* (LEM), which quite convincingly states that P 'things' cannot simultaneously physically exist and not exist ("P or not-P" for every logical proposition P, $A \square \neg A$). Who would dare challenge that tautology of classical logic based on a metaphysical abstraction divorced completely from the self evident facts about the brain dynamics of human beings spelling out its cognitive limitations in the ontological perceptual and epistemological conceptual domains of discourse? What is the rationale behind exclusively investing on the absolute truth of mathematical logic abstractions premised on often convenient and admittedly convincing axioms like LEM? The problema arises from the average observer ignoring the physical reality of a human brain as the main player in co-generating an introspective self search for his identity made possible with the evolution of a language faculty as amply discussed and analyzed elsewhere.* There is a fundamental difference between the role practitioners of professional areas play, e.g., lawyers, clinicians, engineers, etc. in providing real time functional answers to immanent problems challenging the very biopsychosocial equilibrium of real time humans as opposed to the universal goals armed chair academicians, researchers, philosophers have their sights on. Are there two different logics the Sartrean relativism or the radical physic materialistic abstractions? The paradox consists in having both logical approaches simultaneously coexisting in the **same** individual able to engage in deep self introspective but conscious dissociation of immanent emotional self and a transcendental rational self! To harmonize these conflicting strategies we prefer the hybridization strategy of bridging both into an epistemontological existential unit incorporating the best parts of both. We all work best within the set of axiomatic tools we have consciously chosen. Thus the mathematical purists depend more on the symbolic representation of **language** statements whose truth is validated by a set of standard axiomatic logical rules as opposed to **procedural** constructions functionally validated within specific different logic rules for combining the statements, some of which may not even be computable.

The best example of an attempted reconciliation of an informed but ineffable intuition and the tempting truthfulness of LEM was the attempt by L.E.J Brouwer to incorporate the existential experience of **physical** 'change' as monitored by a physical human brain into the **metaphysical** logic symbolism of mathematical abstractions. He concluded in mid 20th. century that mathematical symbolic representations are convenient creations of the mind (we call it the brain) structured for marketing communication purposes among colleagues.

A nutshell, one has the conscious choice of adopting one of two conflicting intuitions about ongoing real time change, either particulate matter is changing, e.g., summating **discontinuous** invisible physical particles into visible sensory realities as falsifiably experienced when a cell (a) divides and forms a visible organ (b) or is **continuous** as our brain also experiences it? Which intuition is correct? The cell (a) is very different form same cell (a') ready to divide by mitosis. Ergo, if (a) then (not a) = (b). Likewise, the human brain, unable to phenomenologically distinguish (a) from (b) retains in living memory the (a) he experienced even when it can be proven otherwise it's no longer there! The invisible change produces the living experience of continuity. Until we reach the potential of a physical description or falsifiable observation experience of change, there is no choice but to affirm the truth of the existential realism, however wrong it may all turn out to be in the future generations, if ever. Which of the two paradoxical intuitions would the reader adopt? Is particulate discontinuous quantum particles more credible than a continuous reality? Could there be a receding physical boundary we can feel comfortable when adopting the abstraction of a set of all sets in existence or do we prefer to adopt a boundless infinite reality poem? What about the equivalent probability of a reciprocal information transfer between transfinite coordinates in n-1 d space time and premotor neocortex phase space mediated by dark baryonic DNA/RNA receptor as posited in our bps model. We even suggested a submodel of a cooperative transfer involving EM and gravitational procession that remains unchallenged? An expansion on the limitation and possibilities of this approach we invite read: http://plato. stanford.edu/entries/intuitionism/#TheCon

SUMMARY AND CONCLUSIONS

For the benefit of more specialized readers we quote from Stanford Encyclopedia of Philosophy."

"The existence of the natural numbers is given by the first act of intuitionism, that is by the perception of a move of time and the falling apart of a life moment into two distinct things: what was, 1, and what is together with what was, 2, and from there to 3, to 4, . . . In contrast to classical mathematics, in intuitionism all infinity is considered to be potential infinity. In particular this is the case for the infinity of the natural numbers. Therefore statements that quantify over this set, such as $(\exists n\, A(n) \vee \neg \exists n A(n))$, have to be treated with caution. On the other hand, the principle of induction is fully acceptable from an intuitionistic point of view . . . . Thus in the context of the natural numbers, intuitionism and classical mathematics have a lot in common. It is only when other infinite sets such as the real numbers are considered that intuitionism starts to differ more dramatically from classical mathematics, and from most other forms of constructivism as well."

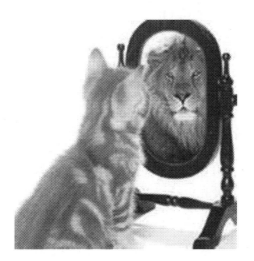

Dr. Angell O. de la Sierra, Esq. In Deltona, Florida Early Winter 2013

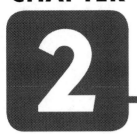

Reflections on the BioPsychoSocial Equilibrium Metaethics

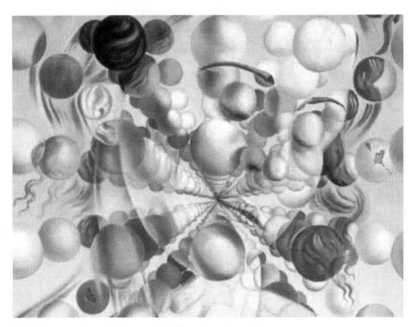

Kantian Art

INTRODUCTION

The current problems of ethical disagreements whether in Washington, DC or the international HiQ community alike surface up because their protagonists may adopt inadequate standards of objectivity. These inadequate standards are subconscious and metaphysical in nature and appeal to the individualized independent reality and truth of biopsychosocio-political (bpsp) survival values in our turf. We are in dire need for objective standards in reasoning to solve practical problems about what to do about real time immanent challenges of existential reality in the real world today and how to avoid probable transcendental predictions tomorrow. If we focus on defining which priorities people reasonably disagree about 'what' to value, we will appreciate the need to reach an agreement about what to do today, here and now, that will also impact what will probably happen tomorrow, somewhere and/or somehow. The priorities are clear, the immanent **present** biopsychosocio-political reality **precedes** any relevant **future** transcendental meta-ethical constructivism and **both** must be guided by normative truths about what one ought to do morally or ethically about either 'economic cliffs' in Washington, DC or a neurophilosophy of consciousness, they both depend on how rational, honest agents (not including politicians for sale) would reason in an idealized deliberative situation.

ARGUMENTATION

Once we deliberately agree on the advantage of starting the analysis with the construction of the 'original position' we would be on our way to find a consensus. This way the practical human problem of disagreement on priority issues should be sufficient, at least in the biopsychosocio-political domain of public discourse, to warrant a stable system of good will cooperation among citizens with different moral, philosophical, and religious views while in their 'original position'. Hopefully, this experience will provide the ground work for at least 'agreements to disagree' on more complex issues of probable transcendental impact in future generations on planet earth or anywhere else. If we can agree on the basic premises of a biopsychosocio-political constructivism where humans are assumed free and equal before any man-made law anywhere according to the principles of justice and respect for the relevant basic institutions of society, then we will be ready for the kind of probable truly meta=ethical constructivism addressing all normative metaphysical and transcendental claims about things like the micro and cosmological transfinities and the corresponding brain dynamic features that must go along with whatever 'agreements to disagree' surge. The big surprise this writer has personally experienced is to realize how difficult it can be to reach hypothetical agreements even among intellectually privileged academicians and researchers who enjoy radically different values and life styles. Was it always that way . . . , can we successfully ignore our gender, religion, moral views, and socio-economic status during a deep introspective search for guiding principles during a 'thought experiment', or is this a sign of the difficult 21st. century times we now experience?

Contrary to the classical Kantian 'practical reason' approach we prefer to account for the nature of moral and normative truths by distinguishing first considerations about the real space-time features of quotidian existential reality of living human species in their ecologically changing environment as preceding their evolution of a rational agency in substantial control of their lives. On this view, reasons for being morally conscious spring from our preceding subconscious BPS needs, interests or desires for survival as a species. As we evolve into maturity beyond the second birthday introspective self consciousness takes root in our nature as evolving rational agents. The subconscious natural forces (genetic, acquired) never cease to play an important, if not decisive, force in our psycho social adult experiences. Every individual and his environmental circumstance has a personal equation representing the degree of ongoing successful evolution towards the Kantian required goal of consciously free willed practical reason and moral obligations to self and others that ideally will become universal and hopefully binding for all rational beings. We do not need to emphasize the great influence a healthy, happy and socially convivial cooperative environment plays into that ongoing evolution towards the practical rational state that makes possible—with the cooperation of the language faculty—the transcendental and reciprocal information transfer in search of species survival answers issues beyond the phenomenologically obvious. These issues vary in complexity and content from the transcendental possible transfinite sources of guidance/righteousness to the immanent solution of the global economic chaos among western nations committed to the freedom and equality of all humans within the liberal democratic socio-political axiological context. Once the 'original position' is freely committed to practical rational judgments can be arrived at, or "constructed," which are likely to be more acceptable to all ordinary citizens regardless of the particular position, race, ethnicity, religion or lifestyle they hold in society and the specific interests that accompany such circumstantial existential realities.

Intuitivism inspired 'constructivism' when applied to transcendental complexities like 'neuro-philosophy of consciousness' or the spontaneous emerging of physical complexity from nothingness or infinities, where self-serving pronouncements are not based on phenomenologically falsifiable observations or measurements or a mathematical logic based epistemology will unfortunately either grounds moral truths on arbitrary self indulging standards, theosophies, materialism, cults, etc. or collapse into a limited realism in its well meant effort to advance our understanding of moral principles and the inherent species cognitive resolution limits. These misguided constructivism rather attempts to create reformist movements that feeds the ego hunger. We prefer to advocate an evolutionary pace congruent, if not in total harmony, with the individualized vital biopsychosocial equilibrium. This is the main reason we prefer a more relaxed 'intuitivistic' mathematical approach different from the classical Kantian model advocating a rational agency wielding strict 'constitutive' standards resisting **any** constructivist effort. So long as there is room for a type of naturalism compatible with the tenets of scientific methodology and metaphysical logic principles in forming our intentions and beliefs, we can make plausible poems about the relevant invisibilities that influence our existence and keep our fingers crossed that our consequent predictions become confirmed by all . . . . sooner or later . . . if ever . . .

Having heretofore argued in behalf of the self evident notion that human phenomenological ontological descriptions and/or the correlative non-physical epistemological explanations are instantiated inside a physical human brain, it is not farfetched to prioritize the biological viability of such physical entity in anticipation of its future ongoing developmental maturation in sensory acuity/resolution before the rest of the body adaptively respond to anything that compromises that biological integrity. A successful defense of that integrity makes possible future brain engagements in its defense against relevant falsifiable objects/ events or experiences outside phenomenological thresholds to detect or even frame into appropriate language symbols to express, e.g., the apparent existence of a non spontaneous and negentropic micro and cosmological order. Neither should it be farfetched to submit that some subhuman creatures share with us the same subconscious concerns for their biological integrity, happiness and cooperative conviviality. If any reader can evidence falsifiable measurements and/or logically credible explanations of subhuman abilities to introspectively search and affirm self as distinct from its surroundings we are all ears. Otherwise we assume this activity as uniquely human. Ergo, the metaphysical carriage cannot precede the physical horse, i.e., epistemology cannot precede ontology as a valid argument to explain the human version of existence and reality. If these premises make any sense, how can the physical brain dynamics make sense of what escapes phenomenological verification or metaphysical logic? Then we make poems and hope the predictions of the wishful thinking model are confirmed by any observer, if ever. The model, theological, scientologist, materialist or otherwise makes its practitioners healthy, happy and accepted by his followers, why not pursue them? It makes existential reality viable like in other advanced subhuman species; if it fulfills your highest aspirations, and makes possible a transitory democratic, free and peaceful society, why give it up? Should we throw the towel and abandon the search for the relevant invisibilities that effectively influence our lives? Never!

Finally, a few notes/guidelines on the evolving practical rationality we tentatively prefer, the 'intuitivistic mathematics' poem challenging the dogma of constitutive rationality 'uber alles' of classical mathematics. The first effort should be directed at dispelling incoherence by adopting and enforcing the 'original position' strategy on the analysts by spelling out clearly the axiological norms that constitute objective and truthful values. Only by engaging in practical reasoning first can produce abstract conceptual norms of universal aspirations. A moral order of values is not discovered but rationally constructed as just normative natural facts that can be investigated by ordinary empirical methods, e.g., polling, constitutional conventions, etc. The mathematical purists should note that this kind of constructivism appealing to norms under the guidelines of practical reason are essentially non-reductive to meaningful parsing symbolism. Likewise a human truth existing outside the activity of a human thinking brain just like an abstract conceptual proposition about an object or event can only become true after the living brain of subject has perceptually experienced its existential structure and/or functional truth. We can extend this argument by proposing that an epistemological deduction/induction can only become false after the living brain of a human subject has subjected the abstraction to appropriate mathematical logic analysis and demonstrated it to be an impossible mental construction, e.g., it is theorized that an average man can swallow an ordinary open umbrella! ☺ Consequently there shouldn't be considered as **human** truths objects or events not yet experienced iff a human subject has **previously** experienced its logical falsehood (by realizing that an appropriate mental construction is not possible).

One of the most controversial and perplexing consequences of intuitionist reasoning is that it is based on the awareness of time as a free will creation of a normal conscious mind, as we often said, a convenient conceptualization of experienced or rationally inferred changes. Like we always said, mathematics are convenient and useful language tools that follow phenomenological existential experiences to begin with. This way present b and past a of same object or event can simultaneously coexist so long as a memory of that past survives the present. This may seem to violate the dogma of the excluded middle, if a then not a (i.e.,

b) is not possible. An extended discussion of this apparent paradox is beyond the scope of this brief introductory presentation.

SUMMARY AND CONCLUSIONS

In this abbreviated summary we have provided arguments in behalf of an intuitionistic model of universal reality which in our BPS model gets tentatively reduced to a human brain based model of an ever changing and evolving existential 4-d space time reality if we objectively consider both the intrinsic limitations and uniqueness of the human phenomenon. Along these admittedly controversial arguments we respectfully challenge several of the time-honored classical conceptualization models of reality in an effort to update its conclusions as justified by reliable modern technological measurements and credible conceptualizations rooted on metaphysical logic. Most of the daring challenges have been based on the undeniable fact that the human cosmology is the product of the human brain activity with all its limitations and uniqueness as argued in 4 published volumes and a treatise on the brain dynamics underlying the neurophilosophy of consciousness.

Dr. Angell O. de la Sierra, Esq. In Deltona, Florida Late Spring 2012.

The Phenomenological Ontological Description or the Constructive Epistemological Explanations of the Real Spatio-temporal Material Beings in 4-d Existential Reality? Metaphysical Idealism or Biopsychosocial (BPS) Realism?

INTRODUCTION

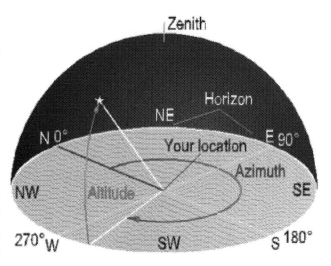

The continuous silent battle for media recognition between practitioners and academicians rages on. Posturing by physicians, psychologists, lawyers and engineers vs. professors, mathematicians, physicists and philosophers looks like the outdated claims of realism exclusivity by Husserl's phenomenology of experienced objective reality vs. equivalent idealism claims by Hilbert's or Mach's metaphysical logic about their subjective symbolic representations thereof. What is ultimately more important, immanent practical or transcendental speculative solutions to guide us today or tomorrow respectively? We think both are just two sides of the same coin and must be considered as such in the proposed dynamic operational algorithm. It integrates both the cooperative inputs of the hands-on lab/clinic practitioners and the arm chair academician brain storms as they evolve into the future in behalf of both the individual and the human species at large. For those of us who have embraced the arguments of quantum theory as an ideal glue to bind the phenomenological with the metaphysical as a way to bring into focus the noumenal structure/function of reality from the invisible extrasensory possibility domain to the credible probable domain. We are still reckoning with the important counterintuitive implications that this binding glue carries. This is especially so when we realize the need for quantum theory to harmonize with general relativity theory which puts the human observer at center stage as should be. But we continue to critically examine why our human species may have no choices but to open new paths as we walk through future unknown fields like the Spanish philosopher Unamuno warned the inquisitive mind: ".caminantes no hay camino, se hace camino al andar." Finding the way across the unknown maze inside a forest is made easier if we admit, albeit tentatively, what appears self evident; we are witnessing a neo-Copernican revolution with the self-conscious human at the center of the universe and advancing with a slow but unrelenting determination to both describe and explain his origins and destiny regardless of his own obvious sense-phenomenal and brain combinatorial limitations in resolving the structure/function features of the diametrically opposite transfinities of the subplanckian and cosmological manifolds. All of this hope is fueled by the information explosion brought about by computerized technology and mathematical sophistication. However, for the existential realist mathematical **possibilities** in abstracto cannot precede physical **probabilities,** just like planning the next step **now** cannot precede dealing with the **future** consequences of the step into new territory yet unmapped; you may praise the abstract Lord but meanwhile pass the real ammunition.

ARGUMENTATION

The diagram above would give the reader the impression that, along the lines of the classical idealism of Hilbert, Mach and others, universal reality can be exclusively reduced to constructive symbolic metaphysical logic symbolisms of purely arithmetical Peano relations that under arbitrary coordinate transformations could be relied upon as the exclusive objective fact of our evolving multiverse. But intuitively we know better that there will be differences in the measurement of e.g., the angle between the two stars, depending on the subjective experience of the observer as it supervenes on the otherwise invariant relationship of the real time observer and the stars. This falsifiable experience incorporates Husserl's phenomenalism and Einstein's general relativity into the algorithm mix. Who should we trust the idealist version or the realist version of existential 4-d reality? The hands-on experimentalist or the armed chair academician? We argue below that both models are incomplete and an objective understanding of human existence requires the synthetic a posteriori synthesis of both, so long as self evident causality principles controls the interpretation. We further speculate how this synthesis is not the final model fitting the human species mesoscopic reality in that it leaves out falsifiable and relevant experiences that resist language description or measurement, existing outside the human threshold for sense-phenomenal or brain combinatorial resolution. But the search continues and we have published a tentative, albeit speculative model of recursive information transfer between our premotor neocortex and the n-1 d spatiotemporal coordinates of an unidentified transfinity source.*

For starters, we all realize that there is more physical content to quotidian, real time existence than sense phenomenal Husserlian reality directly reveals and consequently objective reality cannot be properly studied directly except through the use of appropriate symbols to represent those relevant extrasensory features that are also part and parcel of the experiential present. But, as it happens, the quantum algorithm package also carries along extra classical 'non-locality', arbitrary atomic orbital restrictions like the Leibnitz-Pauli Exclusion Principle, not to mention quantum causality and other non-classical physics relationships between the observation/measurement and the reality witnessed. What cannot be ontologically described as a real space time material being must be epistemologically analyzed and completed by metaphysical symbolic logic construction. As we have repeated so many times, reality is inherently subjective because it is ultimately experienced in the human brain. Consequently appearances based on sense qualities are existentially relevant and an exclusively Newtonian equivalent construction of objective reality in pure analytical geometry symbols is thereby incomplete. We often forget that space and time do not have an independent reality but are necessary constructions of the mind to assign an collectively agreed-upon tempo-spatial location for objects and events in the Leibnitzean sense.

Contrary to the idealism school view, for the newborn to survive to reproductive age s(he) must adapt first to his environmental circumstance by responding with either immediate reflex or a delayed conscious adaptive neuromuscular activity choice as required by metaphysical logic constructs, in that order, i.e., the phenomenological precedes the symbolically inferred as the initiator of the species adaptive responses. One does not construct an objective environment, at any scale, with precise mathematical symbolic coordinates in anticipation of real time users' preferences. It's the other way around where real spatio temporal points reality initiate and guide the symbolic construction of geometrical coordinates. This is not to say that this initial experience expressed in pure symbolic language may thereafter serve as a guide to plan the anticipated future development of a known area. Needless to say, we are in the classical idealistic tradition, formally extrapolating to the very first man in existence acting on strictly inherited sources of information as may still happen in underdeveloped nations. In more developed scenarios it is fair to say that the idealized metaphysical logic model that in principle provides for all known scenarios now constitutes 'proto-factual evidence' to guide and evaluate the worth of new measurements or observations made in the new unknown environment. This way new explanations and subsequent generalizations provide for the evolving new horizons iff the symbolic structure correlates directly with the phenomenological experience.

Contrary to the idealism tradition we believe that the Kantian a priori forms encompassing the totality of our quotidian conscious experiences in our particular ecological niche, e.g., our evolving intuitions about the time and place we cohabit with others, will unavoidably precede any synthetic a posteriori arithmetical model to represent the objective 4-d continuum world construction we aim at when planning for future developments. It's like ideally designing a dynamic jacket fitting all conceivable sizes, shapes, color and preferences as opposed to, once we have experienced the nature of such variations and then using those experiences as a basis on which to design the 'one size fits all' type of solution. Like solving a problem before you know what the problem is, maybe it does not even exist as a reasonable probability.

What it means is that we should not 'substantivate' the required conditions for sense-phenomenal measurements or observations of objects or events to take place. This habit is the major source of categorical confusion between the physical reality of the ideally constructed map and the experienced territory as we so often witness in discussions of complex reality among otherwise privileged minds. Ergo physically empty space-time vacuum is not a territory we can substantiate a priori even by liberating the constraints imposed by numerical metric structures on experienced real time 4-d space time by continuous one-to-one abstract coordinate transformations divorced from existential spacio-temporal reality. If the reader keeps reminding himself that the cognitive capacity of our human species for understanding the meaning of an objective existential reality as a goal exists in a very limited brain capacity for sense-phenomenal and combinatorial resolution, then it should be expected that reality is subjective, emotionally ego centered and existentially guided by reflex intuitions, all of which points to the seeming paradox of a hopefully **invariant** objective goal being relative to the **varying** position in 4-d space time of the individualized observer. This means that relativity is part of the human equation and its influence cannot be effectively and totally neutralized in most humans by the invariance of natural laws and measurable quantities achieved by the mathematical transformations.

The unavoidable co-existence of the phenomenological with the epistemological, as we preach in the biopsychosocial (BPS) model, has to harmonize with experiential causality. Adjectives, verbs and adverbial attributions cannot cause and precede the object or event they are describing in either 4-d existence or anywhere in transfinite space-time unless you want to argue that the Einstenian $E=MC^2$ equivalence is a convenient license to consider energy as immaterial and thus implying/marketing the counter-intuitive existential conclusion/notion that you can get something from nothing. There is nothing wrong with the idealized a priori notions of appearances because material beings in measurable or observed motions need physical boundaries with dimensional coordinates, whether seen or unseen. Consequently we need to characterize that invisible variable container with the x,y,z,t 4-d spatiotemporal dimensions containing mass/energy particles traveling specified linear/curved measurable finite distances in an imposed direction by the gravitational forces of attraction present. The mathematical symbols 'describing' the differential-topological relations of material beings in space time, i.e., the 'logical space' of symbolic arithmetical relations, the structure/ function of an invisible mass, charge, field strength, etc., all of which constitute the required, albeit evolving and tentative, conditions to explain the preceding new experience. The epistemontological hybrid of the BPS model correlates the symbolic structure with experiential reality.

How else can we measure anything moving in any direction without boundaries, experienced or invented? Hilbert and Mach exclusive emphasis on abstract idealism and the opposite physical realism were two extremes that IMHO limited the possibilities of cognitive evolution by denying the possibility of exploring the possibility of n-1d transfinite sources of reciprocal information to explain the self evident order that seems to defy our physical laws of nature, as explained elsewhere in the BPS model of brain dynamics.* If you neglect the existential 4-d territory experience and rely exclusively on the corresponding abstract mapping you will be surprised how the individualized set of real-time circumstantial experiences of the observer (and the observed) will deviate from the theoretical predictions of the mathematical model when navigating in uncharted territories. Expressing it more formally it means that the metric and causal structure of the 4-d real world territory is dynamically evolving before the map catches on, world lines of material points are not rigid straight lines where the inertial, causal and metric structure of the ideal world are impervious to environmental changes, including the position of the theoretical extended human observer. Enter general relativity relevance and the need to harmonize it with quantum probabilities.

Dr. Angell O. de la Sierra, Esq. In Deltona, Florida 11/27/2012

CHAPTER 4

The Need for an Epistemontological Perspective on Existential Reality Analysis

("Clearly there is more to the classical analysis and knowledge of existential reality than the restricted standards of evidence and justification which are most accurately and explicitly represented by metaphysical logic tools and most successfully implemented in the natural sciences." Dr.d)

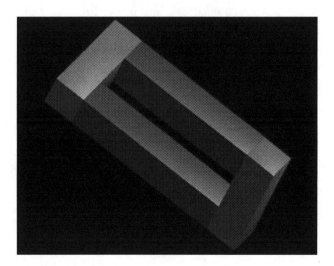

INTRODUCTION

There have been some linguistic purists that have challenged the characterization of our biopsychosocial model of brain dynamics (BPS) as 'epistemontological' and misleading. In Vol. II of "Neurophilosophy of Consciousness, an Epistemontological View of Reality" http://delasierra-sheffer.net/ID7-BPS-info/ID7-BPS-info/index.htm we said: ". . . . Natural language continues to play, in our opinion, a leading role in the formulation and explanation of what is alleged by cosmologists (and other brainy poets) to be a conformation and functioning of the all encompassing global consciousness. We still hope to identify that missing link connecting the sense-phenomenal ontology (of the perceptually falsifiable observations in objects and events, by external or internal sense receptors) and the corresponding abstract epistemology (of the conceptual, mathematical/modal-logic maps) of the experienced existential reality. A tautological, epistemontological hybrid model of reality would be our biggest contribution to the study of consciousness . . . . we had hoped to give a complete ambitious description of the amygdaloid complex as a natural candidate for the seat of consciousness based primarily, among other things, on its well documented participation (with the hippocampus formation) in coordinating the avoidance reflex responses when humans were confronted with natural life-threatening environmental stimuli. This would arguably take care of the ontological aspect of the hybrid model of reality. As it turns out, the stimulating natural object / event in this case is meaning neutral, the semantic tag being provided by inherited life-preserving amygdaloidal audio-visual (and other modalities) codelets as modified by experience. We called the amygdaloidal complex the inherited proto-semantic data base. Pursuant to the analysis, we designated the 'shores' surrounding the Sylvian fissure (perisylvian area) inter-connecting all sensory inputs traveling into Heschl-Wernicke's-angular gyrus region and relaying them to Broca's area (pre-frontal executive cortex), the 'proto-linguistic organ' (plo). We labored hard to weave together a meta-linguistic distributed network headquartered at 'plo' and modeled to integrate nativist considerations on syntax, semantics, referentials, phonology, truth values, pragmatics, vector space network theory and DNA-encoded language inputs. We even thought we had found the 4-d coordinates for Chomsky's generative grammar as the same locus for a regenerative semantics, all embodied by the 'plo'. There we could combine both elements (universal grammar & proto-semantics) and bring to life a comprehensive theory of 'meaning' linking linguistic elements such as figures, signs, noises, marks and body movements as different manifestations of a communication urge, mostly reducible in principle to 'propositional attitudes' as configured in syntax structure and semantics. We hoped it would represent the beginnings of a veritable truth-conditional theory of meaning of high coherence value. We laid the foundations, based on a reinterpretation of Fodor's 'mentalese' and Piaget's theory on language acquisition by the newborn as discussed in Volume I http://delasierra-sheffer.net/ID1-Neurophilo-net/index. htm, chapter 5 and elsewhere. We scattered many seeds on fertile grounds to germinate and flourish but still have not found the magic fertilizer concept to make them sprout into a luxuriant independent existence." We found the classical interpretations of 'ontology' and 'epistemology' too limiting, as if we humans were reacting to different existential realities exclusive of each other and exclusively guided by reason alone. In the classical ontological view arguments excluded un-coded empirical observations of ongoing, real time existential reality in our 4-d space time reality where emotions often play a decisive role and were instead arguments for the conclusion that God exists, from almost exclusively 'rational' analytic a-priori premises and 'objective' scriptures sources to sustain it. Sometimes important and relevant, self evident and falsifiable information from vital experiences are ineffable and resist conventional linguistic formulation or coding; are they predictable object and/or future events acquired by revelations?

Likewise, classical epistemology focuses on the reliability of classical information sources in the generation of knowledge and justified beliefs in their perceptual descriptions or inferred explanations. When concerned for the necessary and sufficient conditions of knowledge they are only considering the classical sense-phenomenal or metaphysical logic representation sources where their structure and limitations are spelled out. The characterization as a justified belief is limited to rational sources amenable to analytic or synthetic tools examination not including emotionally-laden or ineffable intuitions that resist their framing into conventional linguistic formulations for communication purposes. And we ask, why should they be epistemologically ignored as a justifiable source? Epistemology is ultimately about the creation and communication of ALL knowledge that is relevant to the health, happiness and social conviviality of ALL living humans regardless of the source.

We then concluded: "The solution is a synthesis of the falsifiable empirical descriptions with the mathematical logic explanations using the metaphysical tool of quantum theory. This synthetic amalgamation of the perceptual and the conceptual required no less than a modification of both quantum theory and classical logic to accommodate the human 'free will' between the indeterministic epistemological explanations and the ontological descriptions of a probable world. Enter the epistemontological model successes and pitfalls as described below". We now expand further on the justifications for this approach for the benefit of my detractors.

ARGUMENTATION

The most important philosophical issues about the human species existential reality, life and consciousness, lie at the triangular intersection of logic, epistemology and ontology. We never understood why these diverse fields within philosophy could not come together as one single philosophical problem when restricted to the discussion of the human species survival in the real time 4-d mesoscopic world. To realize this goal we have to give a corresponding reinterpretation about their inevitable co-relations between them forming what we have called an 'epistemontological hybrid'. In this response article we will provide the argument/ justifications for such—not so novel—approach if we analytically examine the human species condition in its consistent existential goal of attaining biological health, psychic happiness and social acceptance among our contemporary peers, i.e., BPS approach. We will stress where logic, epistemology and ontology overlap as a 'living' unit.

We realize that the premises we offer are themselves questionable but we invite anyone able to provide a more objective and credible model. We are talking about the same entity (individualized human being) living in a constantly challenging and changing ecosystem not necessarily consciously chosen/controlled by him according to biological and psycho-social imperatives/drives for self preservation against the body proper and external environmental demands for adaptive solution. Ongoing existential reality is one and exists in the individualized human brain. We argue about different aspects of same human entity and his circumstance which is **not** the same as when differences involve contentious philosophical ideas such as essence, concept, and meaning such as genetic memory endowment largely under unconscious control, acquired memory experiences largely under subconscious control and most importantly, the ability to make self-conscious choices from existing alternatives with the cooperation of the language machinery as detailed elsewhere. Our approach has important epistemological elements of scientific realism when including the content of our best theories and models about both observable and unobservable aspects of the perceptual/ sense phenomenal world described by science methodology without excluding relevant metaphysical and semantic dimensions. It makes no intuitive sense to deny that the ongoing human existential reality is both brain and mind-dependent, i.e., no brain, no conscious mind reality. Why believe that relevant, consistent and important human experiences that cannot be directly observed or measured because of their sub-threshold phenomenal invisibility cannot exist? Why throw in the towel instead of attempting analytical and/or synthetic a-priori/a-posteriori symbolic or sentential representations and extract their epistemological and semantic probability content? Representation problems can be adequately managed by assigning probability scales on their different types. Sense-phenomenal and falsifiable descriptions of experienced objects/events by normal persons under similar circumstances that generate predictable and falsifiable events, including fMRI neuronal activation of otherwise normal subjects of different language backgrounds top the list of reliable beliefs; especially when mathematical logic principles are used, like the 'law of the excluded middle'. It is much more difficult to consider sub clinical/sub threshold disease manifestations (inherited or acquired) whether subconscious or conscious and deliberately non ethical or amoral. Arguably, these objective controls would take care of conceptual schemes consciously adopted or not. Unfortunately even judgments rooted on model theoretic models carefully controlling all of known indeterministic variables may still be wrong because of the subthreshold dimension of ongoing evolutionary changes in structure and/or function of objects or events under consideration. Last but not least stands the most controversial aspect of the BPS equilibrium model good for any animal and human species in the most primitive state. We have also argued that, thanks to the exclusively human species capacity to introspectively co-generate a self conscious state and thought with the cooperation of an inner language, humans can transcend the subconscious state of other subhumans and linked/ entangled with undefined transfinite sources of information and guidance in behalf of the species survival thereby adding a new metaphysical logic dimension to explain the apparent violation of the entropic natural laws that require that the micro and macro complex self evident order we witness cannot be spontaneous lest we revise the natural laws we so much revere. The 'intelligent designer' postulate, whatever, whenever or however manifested is required by metaphysical logic analysis and needs no support from theological arguments. This is the best argument we can market about the serious sense-phenomenal (internal body proper and external) and brain combinatorial conceptual limitations of our human species. We are fully aware of the difficulty of accepting the premise about the cogeneration of language and thought as mediated by the proto language machinery and detailed elsewhere. This way we can communicate to ourselves and others and also achieve the introspective self-conscious state so important in freely willing the best adaptive solution to familiar and new contingencies in the environment that may pose a challenge to the BPS equilibrium dynamics of the ongoing human being or, in addition, consciously negating ourselves self preservation in the altruistic behalf of others. In this respect Wittgenstein provided, in our opinion, a metaphysical "language game" tool with its own individualized criteria for justification by adopting a particular solution tailored to the immediate and/or transcendental needs of the decision maker, one best suited to his particular needs and conveniences, i.e., his existential circumstances (genetic, acquired, etc). This opens the door to subconscious or conscious individualized circumstances, consciously willed or imposed (emotions, disease, deprivations, natural intelligence, etc.) where natural theology, materialism, cults or other forms of beliefs naturally thrive because we need to satisfy the innate drive to explain our origins and destiny according to our intellectual resources and existential experiences. Consequently the Judeo-ChrIslamic "language game" would model the best explanation of the relevant, consistent and falsifiable experiences of the sense-phenomenal invisibilities outside their perceptual threshold for scientific physical characterization and outside the 4-d space time of our existential reality, yet essential as they are at either end of the dimensional spectrum, from the sub-Planckian to the cosmological levels of organization. Organized religious beliefs, including the materialist physicalist faith or equivalent cults depend on recorded or embellished historical 'facts' such as the Judeo-ChrIslamic scriptures or other convenient falsifiable experience during the normal, diseased or self-induced hallucinatory mind state. What is important for the preservation of the human species viability is to achieve, maintain and sustain a state of biopsychosocial equilibrium as evolution slowly changes the survival scenario where the metaphysical commitment of the 'religious belief' as expressed in the language game credo is consistent with cooperative psychosocial survival during the ongoing and quotidian existential living in mesoscopic reality. It should be noticed that the language game does not exclude serious intellectual enquiry of the curious mind. So we now suggest a new type of 'constructive empiricism' by substituting the classical epistemological view that rejects as credible anything unobservable that scientific theories model.

Finally, one additional caveat concerning the 'language game' as when the rules of grammar are forced into a mathematical logic straight jacket. We have detailed the Fodorian 'propositional attitude' representations elsewhere. They are meant to cogently express human attitudes on beliefs, doubts, sorrows, etc. whose information content is true or false and possesses modal properties such as being necessary, possible or contingent but, we ask, are they still fit to accommodate the expression of factual, abstract, real or imagined entities effectively and still remain propositions?

Many of the problems about the reliability and flexibility of linguistic representations of observed or inferred existential experiences have been solved by the adoption of 'Bayesian epistemology' that essentially extends the certainty constraints of deductive logic of mathematical representations to the probable inferences of inductive logic, i.e., extends the justification of the laws of deductive logic to include a justification for the laws of inductive logic by adopting probabilistic and coherence criteria, what is called conditional probability or degrees of confidence. A coherence theory of **truth, knowledge or justification** supposes that the **truth** of any (true) proposition consists in its coherence with some specified set of propositions.

SUMMARY AND CONCLUSIONS

All things relevant, being hopefully considered above, we prefer to stick to the core concepts of common sense, the importance of individualizing the conclusions on the BPS needs and conveniences of the unit, human being singularity before doing extrapolations about the average unit. Just like considerations on space and time causation, we need to include other relevant non-classical aspects of meaning, reference and truth as discussed. Their relevance should not have to be earned by the reduction of the non-classical sources of information to an allegedly more basic, secure and convenient realm of concepts, e.g., based exclusively on factual experience as represented by symbolic and/or sentential logic language. After all, as Newman pointed out: ". . . . people made up their minds on non-religious issues and argue that by the same standards religious beliefs were justified." As a result, he qualified evidentialism by insisting that "an *implicit* and *cumulative* argument could lead to justified certainty." Perceptual 'facts' always have an embodiment whether they are veridical, illusory or the result of hallucinations. Part of this problem is that mathematics is incorrectly regarded as a science even though observations or measurements of objects/events existing in space time do not mediate in their symbolic or sentential representations of their structure and functions, useful as they indeed are when making projections into probable future scenarios. In other words, the specific deduction from basic principles that characterize the mathematical methods of investigation is very different from the inductive methods of investigation in the natural sciences aimed at acquiring just general knowledge and consequently tend to be less certain and more susceptible to revision than the corresponding mathematical theories derived therefrom. For these reasons, the materialistic physicalist faith or belief poses serious problems of reliability and certainty, not very different from the equivalent problems in theological beliefs. As Kant's realism pointed out in his "Critique of Pure Reason", existential realism brings in many more variables into relevant consideration than the classical sciences. As Spanish philosopher Ortega y Gasset pointed out "Every opinion is a theoretical argument" because all epistemological theories of judgment should bring together ALL relevant fundamental issues: e.g., semantics, logic, psychology, ontology, and action theory. Any theory of human rationality must consider the capacity for judgment of the individualized human mind after carefully examining the propositional content of an expressed judgment, especially its relative content of sense-phenomenal and *transcendental idealism* experiences. Not an easy examination for a psychiatric practitioner!

Clearly there is more to the analysis and knowledge of existential reality than the restricted standards of evidence and justification which are most accurately and explicitly represented by metaphysical logic tools and most successfully implemented in the natural sciences. This applies to all branches of knowledge and all tools of enquiry. We have tried an epistemontological approach where the classic metaphysical tool of ontological deduction from basic principles derived from all forms of inductive epistemological enquiries about all sources of relevant information becomes a veritable transformation of absolute presuppositions controlling heuristic principles. This hybridization stimulates the identification of foundational knowledge of reliable premises or first truths on which to base our conceptualizations about existential reality. It also allows for the inclusion of evolutionary processes modifying the perceptual and conceptual informational profiles accruing as a function of unavoidable spatiotemporal changes. This may even stimulate further study into the claim that there exist abstract mathematical 'objects' whose existence is independent of us and our language, thought, and practices and even the possibility of the logical interaction between theology, law, science and social history.

5 The Phenomenological Ontological Description or the Constructive Epistemological Explanations of the Real Spatio-temporal Material Beings in 4-d Existential Reality? Metaphysical Idealism or Biopsychosocial (BPS) Realism?

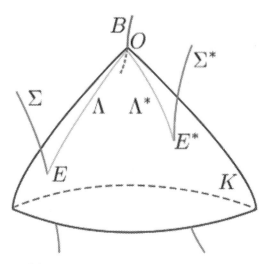

Angular distance δ between two stars observed by O, absolute or relative?

INTRODUCTION

The continuous silent battle for media recognition between practitioners and academicians rages on. Posturing by physicians, psychologists, lawyers and engineers vs. professors, mathematicians, physicists and philosophers looks like the outdated claims of **realism** exclusivity by Husserl's phenomenology of experienced objective reality vs. equivalent **idealism** claims by Hilbert's or Mach's metaphysical logic about their subjective symbolic representations thereof. What is ultimately more important, immanent **practical** or transcendental **speculative** solutions to guide us today or tomorrow respectively? We think both are just two sides of the same coin and must be considered as such as the proposed dynamic operational algorithm integrates both the cooperative inputs of the hands-on lab/clinic practitioners and the arm chair academician brain storms evolve into the future in behalf of both the individual and the human species at large. For those of us who have embraced the arguments of quantum theory as an ideal glue to bind the phenomenological with the metaphysical as a way to bring into focus the noumenal structure/function of reality from the invisible extrasensory possibility domain to the credible probable domain, we are still reckoning with the important counterintuitive nature this binding glue carries. This is especially so when we realize quantum theory's need to harmonize with general relativity theory which puts the human observer at center stage as should be. But we continue to critically examine why our human species may have no choices but to open new paths as we walk through future unknown fields like the Spanish philosopher Unamuno warned the inquisitive mind: ".caminantes no hay camino, se hace camino al andar." Finding the way across the unknown maze is made easier if we admit, albeit tentatively, what appears self evident; we are witnessing a neo-Copernican revolution with the self-conscious human at the center of the universe with a slow but unrelenting determination to both describe and explain his origins and destiny regardless of his own obvious sense-phenomenal and brain combinatorial limitations in resolving the structure/function features of the diametrically opposite transfinities of the subplanckian and cosmological manifolds. All of this thanks to the information explosion brought about by computerized technology. For the existential realist mathematical possibilities in abstracto cannot precede physical probabilities, just like planning the new next step cannot precede dealing with the new consequences of the step into new territory yet unmapped; you may praise the abstract Lord but meanwhile pass the real ammunition.

ARGUMENTATION

The diagram above would give the reader the impression that, along the lines of the classical idealism of Hilbert, Mach and others, universal reality can be exclusively reduced to constructive symbolic metaphysical logic symbolisms of purely arithmetical relations that under arbitrary coordinate transformations could be relied upon as the exclusive objective fact of our evolving multiverse. But intuitively we know better that there will be differences in the measurement of the angle between the two stars depending on the **subjective experience** of the observer as it supervenes on the otherwise invariant relationship of the real time observer and the stars. This falsifiable experience incorporates Husserl's phenomenalism and Einstein's general relativity into the algorithm mix. Who should we trust the **idealist** version or the **realist** version of existential 4-d reality? The hands-on experimentalist or the armed chair academician? We argue below that both models are incomplete and objective understanding of human existence requires the synthetic a posteriori synthesis of both, so long as self evident causality principles controls the interpretation. We further speculate how this synthesis is not the final model fitting the human species mesoscopic reality in that it leaves out falsifiable and relevant experiences that resist language description or measurement, existing outside the human threshold for sense-phenomenal or brain combinatorial resolution. But the search continues and we have published a tentative, albeit speculative model of recursive information transfer between our premotor neocortex and the n-1 d spatiotemporal coordinates of an unidentified transfinity source.*

For starters, we all realize that there is more content to quotidian, real time existence than sense phenomenal Husserlian reality directly reveals and consequently objective reality cannot be properly studied directly except through the use of appropriate symbols to represent those relevant extrasensory features that are also part and parcel of the experiential present. But, as it happens, the quantum algorithm package also carries along extra classical 'non-locality', arbitrary atomic orbital restrictions like the Leibnitz-Pauli Exclusion Principle, not to mention quantum causality and other non-classical physics relationships between the observation/measurement and the reality witnessed. What cannot be ontologically described as a real space time material being must be epistemologically analyzed and completed by metaphysical symbolic logic construction. As we have repeated so many times, reality is inherently subjective because it is ultimately experienced in the human brain. Consequently appearances based on sense qualities are existentially relevant and an exclusively Newtonian equivalent construction of objective reality in pure analytical geometry symbols is thereby incomplete. We often forget that space and time do not have an independent reality but are necessary constructions of the mind to assign an collectively agreed-upon tempo-spatial location for objects and events in the Leibnitzean sense. Contrary to the idealism school view, for the newborn to survive to reproductive age s(he) must adapt first to his environmental circumstance by responding with either **immediate** reflex or **delayed** conscious adaptive neuromuscular activity choices as required by metaphysical logic constructs, in that order, i.e., the phenomenological precedes the symbolically inferred as the initiator of the species adaptive responses. One does not construct an objective environment, at any scale, with precise mathematical symbolic coordinates in anticipation of real time users' preferences. It's the other way around where real spatio temporal points reality initiate and guide the symbolic construction of geometrical coordinates. This is not to say that this initial experience expressed in pure symbolic language may thereafter serve as a guide to plan the anticipated future development of a known area. Needless to say we are, in the classical idealistic tradition, formally extrapolating to the very first man in existence acting on strictly inherited sources of information as may still happen in underdeveloped nations. In more developed scenarios it is fair to say that the idealized metaphysical logic model that in principle provides for all **known** scenarios now constitutes 'proto-factual evidence' to guide and evaluate the worth of new measurements or observations made in the new unknown environment. This way new explanations and subsequent generalizations provide for the evolving new horizons iff the symbolic structure correlates directly with experience.

Contrary to the idealism tradition we believe that the Kantian a priori forms encompassing the totality of our quotidian conscious experiences in our particular ecological niche, e.g., our evolving intuitions about the time and place we cohabit with others, will unavoidably precede any synthetic a posteriori arithmetical model to represent the objective 4-d continuum world construction we aim at when planning for future developments. It's like ideally designing a dynamic jacket fitting all conceivable sizes, shapes, color and preferences as opposed to, once we have experienced the nature of such variations and then using those experiences as a basis on which to design the 'one size fits all' type of solution. Like solving a problem before you know what the problem is, maybe it does not even exist as a reasonable probability. What it means is that we should not 'substantivate' the required conditions for sense-phenomenal measurements or observations of objects or events to take place. This habit is the major source of categorical confusion between the physical reality of the ideally constructed map and the experienced territory as we so often witness in discussions of complex reality among otherwise privileged minds. Ergo physically empty space-time vacuum is **not** a territory we can substantivate a priori even by liberating the constraints imposed by numerical metric structures on experienced real time 4-d space time by continuous one-to-one abstract coordinate transformations divorced from existential spacio-temporal reality. If the reader keeps reminding himself that the cognitive capacity of our human species for understanding the meaning of an objective existential reality as a goal exists in a very limited brain capacity for sense-phenomenal and combinatorial resolution, then it should be expected that reality is subjective, emotionally ego centered and existentially guided by reflex intuitions, all of which points to the seeming paradox of a hopefully **invariant** objective goal being **relative** to the position in 4-d space time of the individualized observer. This means that relativity is part of the human equation and its influence cannot be effectively and totally neutralized in most humans by the invariance of natural laws and measurable quantities achieved by the mathematical transformations.

The unavoidable co-existence of the phenomenological with the epistemological, as we preach in the BPS model, has to harmonize with experiential causality. Adjectives, verbs and adverbial attributions cannot cause and precede the object or event they are describing in 4-d existence or anywhere in transfinite space-time unless you want to argue that the Einstenian $E=MC^2$ equivalence is a convenient license to consider energy as immaterial and thus implying/marketing the counter-intuitive existential conclusion/notion that you can get something from nothing. There is nothing wrong with the idealized a priori notions of appearances because material beings in measurable or observed motions need physical boundaries with dimensional coordinates, whether seen or unseen. Consequently we need to characterize that invisible variable container with the x,y,z,t 4-d spatiotemporal dimensions containing mass/energy particles traveling specified linear/curved measurable finite distances in an imposed direction by gravitational forces of attraction present. The mathematical symbols 'describing' the differential-topological relations of material beings in space time, i.e., the logical space of symbolic arithmetical relations, the structure/function of an invisible mass, charge, field strength, etc., all of which constitute the required, albeit evolving and tentative, conditions to explain the preceding new experience. The epistemontological hybrid of the BPS model correlates the symbolic structure with experiential reality.

How else can we measure anything moving in any direction without boundaries, experienced or invented? Hilbert and Mach exclusive emphasis on abstract idealism and the opposite physical realism were two extremes that IMHO limited the possibilities of cognitive evolution by denying the possibility of exploring the possibility of n-1d transfinite sources of reciprocal information to explain the self evident order that seems to defy our physical laws of nature, as explained elsewhere in the BPS model of brain dynamics.* If you neglect the existential 4-d territory experience and rely exclusively on the corresponding abstract mapping you will be surprised how the individualized set of real-time circumstantial experiences of the observer will deviate from the theoretical predictions of the mathematical model when navigating in uncharted territories. Expressing it more formally it means that the metric and causal structure of the 4-d real world territory is dynamically evolving before the map catches on, world lines of material points are not rigid straight lines where the inertial, causal and metric structure of the ideal world are impervious to environmental changes, including the position of the theoretical extended human observer. Enter general relativity relevance and the need to harmonize it with quantum probabilities.

*< http://delasierra-sheffer.net/ID6-Internet-wz/Treatise%20final%20version.pdf>

Dr. Angell O. de la Sierra, Esq. In Deltona, Florida 11/27/2012

6 Is Human Existential Reality Discovered or Invented? Determined or Consciously Free Willed?

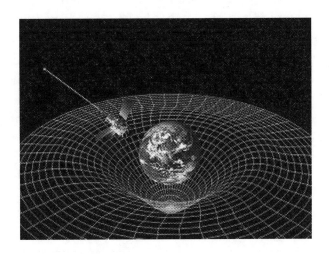

INTRODUCTION

<u>Immanuel Kant</u> does not need my defense but many years have passed since he presented solid arguments in defense of the **ontological** approach of science methodology when he suggested that the familiar 3-d cage life we humans experience in our quotidian existence was an **inevitable** consequence of the **epistemologically** derived inverse square <u>law of universal gravitation,</u> in that order. Yet, we read about recent arguments by the likes of Feyerabend (See his "Tyranny of Science") taking the opposite extreme view that ontological measurements and observations are incomplete and the conclusions derived therefrom not better than self-serving biases projecting a monolithic and unfounded 'world view' of reality. On the other extreme we find <u>John D. **Barrow</u> who in 2004 argued that it is the other way around, that it is the 'ontological fact' of an inferred three-dimensionality of space, in that order, that explains why we see inverse-square force laws in Nature. We continue to argue that those extreme views are unnecessary if we accept the 4 essential premises of our human species existential reality inside our 4-d Minkowsky spacetime cage: 1) human species self

evident sensory and brain combinatorial limitations, 2) reality is in our brains, 3) perceptual attributions of material objects and events do not have an independent reality outside the mass or its motions that makes their description possible, regardless of our inability to always measure its mass (what) or specify its space coordinates (where) at any given time (when). Finally it would seem as if 4) our species, besides its perceptual anatomical limitation to a 4-d space time sensory world, our brain is also constrained to process environmental non linear sensory information input when linearized by sensory receptor activity and language processing.

It is difficult for most readers to understand and appreciate the special gift of the language machinery that makes it possible to articulate and communicate how we can ontologically **describe** what our external and body proper receptors experience and epistemologically **explain** the relevant, ever present but invisible objects and events beyond the sensory threshold to be described. Ergo, the need for a hybrid epistemontological biopsychosocial (BPS) model of reality which we argue should be rooted on the quantum theoretical probabilities of their prediction being measured directly or indirectly. To follow, we offer more arguments in defense of this brain dynamics model which still requires a complete harmony between the quantized and the relativistic, seemingly continuous reality. Does that mean we should stop investigating that transfinite invisible source of inspiration/information that makes possible the historical evolutionary and negentropic path of the human race that defies natural laws? We cannot even avoid that genetic drive fueling our species to search for an explanation of its genesis and eschatological destiny.

ARGUMENTS

Most people may have not watched carefully how a spinning top toy rotates clockwise on its vertical axis (poles) when observed moving on a 2-d plane glass surface table. It's location in space is easily determined from the address of the house where the table is located. As it spin/rotates about its vertical axis we notice that it may also revolve around describing an elliptical path easy to represent on a planar x,y grid diagram on the table surface. But it also shows precession movements about same axis of rotation as it slows down. Since the top is not flat we can conveniently imagine it being spherical and its axis a third dimension 'z' perpendicular to the table surface axis before it slowed down and precession started. We can now see from the **observation** that the solid spinning top is best represented as a hollow volumetric sphere in motion in 3-d space x,y,z. were it not for the pull of gravity that constrains the spinning movement to a 2-d surface, planar or curved if I imagine the table surface as deformed. When the observer looks down (e.g., with a flash light shining down from above the table) he will notice the north polar end of the vertical axis as it spins clockwise in relation to the axis but counterclockwise if the south polar end is now observed from under the transparent table, looking upwards. Which alternative would your 'absolute' description favor? If the spherical spinning top were the earth sphere and the flash light were the sun we would have to incline the light 90 degrees from the imaginary vertical axis so that 'sun will appear' as if moving east → west. With your left thumb pointing up try rotating it along your curved fingers clockwise. Now incline your thumb 'axis' until you reach 90 degrees and think about the new horizontal axis position in respect to the fixed sun above, etc. Continue until you complete 180 degrees when thumb points down; and you will observe the rotation of fingers is now counterclockwise as you look down, same as if you had looked up when viewing from under the table! You intuitively conclude, with Einstein, that the **ontological** description depends on the 'relative' position of the observer in respect to the moving object being described.

Notice also that the analysis depends on the spinning top never slowing down because if it did the original vertical polar axis will incline and precessional movement of the spherical axis will be seen as it rotates on its axis. Now you can predict that if the polar axis inclination were 90 degrees from the vertical (instead of the measured 27 degrees inclination of the earth), then, as your left thumb 'north polar axis' approaches east (90 degrees), your hand rotation will see the **direct** rays from the 'stationary' flash light (sun) rising north and setting south! Can we make predictions if we were to observe in nature significant earth changes in that direction, e.g., earth rotation is slowing down and it takes >24 hours to repeat a day-night cycle, earth axis inclination is increasing, sunset is becoming a southern spectacle, etc. Can we now start describing the human species eschatological end of times when rotation will come to a stop as we bake at solar oven temperatures before the sun reaches its peak temperatures,., etc., etc.? Armageddon?

Furthermore, an observer can at will **measure** the time it takes for any point 'a' (e.g., jet airlines) on the surface of any convenient sphere (e.g., the earth) to complete a full rotation and return to the same location point of observation (e.g., Los Angeles, California). Or assume the jet airlines flying eastward and landing on point 'b' (e.g., New York City longitude). It is not surprising how much simpler it would be to, based on those ontological measurements, how one can epistemologically infer that if the spinning top were a spherical object rotating or in precession about its polar axis one could accurately predict, based on this model, the **probability** of any point on that surface to complete a full cycle in a given time or the probability of point 'a' traveling to another point 'b' in a given time; providing that the point is moving at uniform velocity (not accelerating). At present that trip eastward from Los Angeles to New York City can be completed in < one hour as predicted when traveling at non-uniform velocities, i.e., accelerating! Likewise, the epistemontological hybrid model based on falsifiable observations conceptualizes reality (sub atomic or cosmological) as being contained/bound inside a Riemann sphere where predictions are made possible by quantum probabilistic considerations. This is true whether the sphere represents the sub-Planckian or the cosmological scale. One thing is clear, the ontological observation was experienced in a 4-d space time manifold assisted by epistemological explanations based on metaphysical logic we conveniently used to represent the invisible but relevant object or event physically experienced directly or objectively/logically so implied. This implied hybrid approach has been the most successful 'science' our species has relied on and enjoyed its technological consequences.

Should we then be surprised that, based on previous observations on the <u>flux</u> behavior of 3-d solids under the influence of a gravitational field of measurable strength made possible the reduction of the observation as the result of the operation of an <u>inverse-square law</u> as Kant had suggested? After all nobody has ever witnessed apples falling upwards toward the clouds under the influence of earth gravity pull according to the predictions of the inverse square law. This is not to say that according to that same model the apple could also ascend upwards if **all** its particles had simultaneously, at one point in time, same spin up configuration, an event of extremely low probability in existential reality. Epistemological models of **experienced** unfamiliar contingencies, especially when they escape sensory/instrumental detection, are based on analogies from relevant **previous** related empirical observations. Once this experience is recorded in memory then our intellect can make predictions based on the model, in that order. One can imagine anyone trying to account for almost an infinite number of dimensional observations without having a model that provides a common denominator to all, at the expense of absolute certainty. The uncertainty is unavoidable for the species because of the perceptual/conceptual limitations described. Consequently, we also have to be aware about the added constraints the model may provide, e.g., the extremes of negative and positive infinities in size/dimension, from the receding pre-Planckian sub-atomic to the expanding cosmological dimensions. Enter renormalizations and unreal abstract assumptions to reduce the number of simultaneous variables in operation.

These are the super complex examples of cases where the mathematical logic controls the ontological observation as we see in projective geometry where we must avoid models that approach either zero or infinity values because those values cannot be measured and consequently are meaningless in real time quotidian existence. To illustrate, this may well be the case when we realize that, e.g., two 3-d spheres of radius 'r' each having a surface area $= 4\pi r^2$ where the strength of the <u>gravitational fields</u> pull between their two bodies when separated by a distance of r would be inversely proportional to r^{N-1}. As Kant suggested, this is consequent to the presence of a gravitational force acting as predicted by the <u>inverse-square law</u> and by the concept of <u>flux</u> relating the proportional relationship of flux density and the strength of the gravitational field. If $N = 3$, then 3-dimensional solid objects have surface areas proportional to the square of their size, i.e., a sphere of <u>radius</u> r has area of $4\pi r^2$. The important theoretical anticipation comes when considering any space of N dimensions separating any two bodies 'a','b', sub-atomic or cosmological, the strength of the gravitational pull between the two bodies separated by a distance of r would be inversely proportional to r^{N-1}. Consider the magic scenario when N=1 unit dimension and 'r'=0 or when dealing with negative dimensions and their square roots that give rise to imaginary numbers!

As some HiQers sometimes believe, space time is not distorted because of gravitational attraction by a massive body because space time is massless. Instead, the curved distorsion imposed on a plane surface is just a representation of the <u>coordinate system</u> grid lines predicted to be followed by an independent massive object moving along those lines when under the influence of the <u>gravity</u> pull. The alert reader should have noticed how the existential sensory **discovery** of 'change' as being essentially **experienced** as linear-forward and the discovery of how this 'change' varies depending on the relative positions of the observer and the changing object/event **precedes** the conceptualization of time as linear-forward and how relativity rules explains the trajectory of objects in space motion. Time, unlike empirical 'change', is not an independent variable advancing at a fixed rate in all <u>reference frames</u> as demonstrated by the measured "<u>time dilation</u>" observed when measured time (not change) slowed down at higher speeds of the reference frame relative to another reference frame as explained in the theory of "<u>special relativity</u>". With the **invention** of 'time' as a <u>fourth dimension</u> to be incorporated into our planar or spherical <u>Euclidean space</u> perspective of an <u>universe</u> with a three <u>dimensions</u> coordinate system, it was now possible to thereby create a single <u>manifold</u> that makes it possible to understand the complex workings of existential reality at the mesoscopic, <u>supergalactic</u> and <u>subatomic</u> levels of organization. Welcome 'spacetime' invention. I am only asking for the same consideration when reviewing my conceptualization of reciprocal, transcendental information transfer between transfinity and premotor human neocortical phase space.

Fortunately for the environment, our human species are passive actors/witnesses before the grandeur of the supergalactic/cosmological level where we have invented the concept of a single abstract <u>universe</u> or <u>manifold</u> consisting of observable "events" (what) whose location (where) is described by some type of <u>coordinate system</u> as it happens (when) without being able to control or influence as yet its course of events. In the cosmological domain there are no objects small enough to suffer physical modifications (shape, size, color, etc.) or in any other way be subject to our human manipulations to alter their evolutionary progression, only abstract dimensionless or massless singularity points that some feverish minds also invent to react with discovered objective reality . . . . and sometimes get away with it!

Thus we invent the <u>latitude</u> and <u>longitude</u> abstractions for location, time to describe the perceptual changes observed in the ever present <u>events</u> until we run into logical cul de sacs, especially when, in pursuing our zeal to unify different systems, we find restrictions in the use of common dimensions, e.g., relativity and quantum coordinate dimensions. But dimensions should not be understood as physical attributes of space but just as components of the coordinate grid system when undergoing <u>coordinate transformations</u>. As it may turn out to be, if we are successful in unifying general relativity with quantum theory by considering all of existential reality, of any measurable dimension or not, as contained inside bound hollow spheres of varying radius, e.g., a Riemannian sphere, will arguably dispense of any renormalization or compactifying effort as argued elsewhere. As it stands, dimensions beyond the real time 4-d mesoscopic coordinate space or 'superspace' would only appear to make a difference at the <u>subatomic</u> level if the reconciliation effort is successful and quantum gravity is accepted. This effort in formulating a credible theory exhibiting <u>supersymmetry</u> is mind boggling and requires harmonizing the 'bosonic' 4-d degrees of freedom in real numbers with the <u>fermionic</u> 'anticommuting imaginary dimensions' (<u>Grassmann numbers</u>) and its multiple degrees of freedom. The long range predictions of this <u>particular mathematical model</u> will provide the best veritable science fiction script . . . if nothing else!

Yet, this far-fetched hybrid epistemontological supermodel, contrary to extreme materialism and/or theology equivalents (e.g., 'cults') cannot be ever convincing to the vast majority of individuals populating our special planet earth because the human species is known to be genetically driven to unconsciously protect and sustain a biological integrity, memory driven to subconsciously experience and prefer psychic well being and happiness by triggering an armamentarium of neuro-hormonal tools that renders them, in addition, capable of sharing in social conviviality, depending on their individualized biopsychosocial (BPS) past experiences and circumstances which determines which element is in control of their overt behavior, exclusive self indulgence, exclusive altruism or a healthy balance of healthy, ethical/moral and convivial personality in equilibrium with ongoin, real time existential reality (BPS equilibrium). Recorded history testifies to the truth of such types at all times.

But this BPS equation of brain dynamics would be incomplete if we were to negate the self-evident existential curiosity we humans experience about our species genesis and eschatological destiny which we are able to report thanks to the uniquely human ability for introspective self search and the expression of the results via the also unique 'inner' or verbally reported language machinery. This is the realm of consciousness as another dimension beyond the mesoscopic 4-d, quotidian existential reality into the unknown supercomplexity of an invisible transfinity beyond the scope of scientific ontological and brain metaphysical logic resolution for certainty. So we write poetry and formulate convenient theologies that satisfy all unavoidable believer, from the extremes of materialism to the extremes of mysticism and organized religions in between. We have no other choices because of the anatomico-physiological, ecological and cosmological circumstances that condition and modify our behavior.

Prudence and wisdom tells us that there is **not** in existence for believers a charted path to walk with certainty, that we **individually** have to make the path as we walk hopefully with the benefit of a biopsychosocial equilibrium as defined, like the famous Spanisher philosopher said "Caminantes, no hay camino, se hace camino al andar" which I would complete by warning about the roughness and obstacles to be found during the walk, "Hacia las estrellas por asperos senderos" or in Latin "Ad Astra per Asperas". Emmanuel Kant exemplifies this strategy walking along a path criticizing an exclusive pure reason protocol to avoid the temptations of the extreme materialistic believers (some scientists and philosophers) and the temptations of the extreme mystic believers (cults, etc.). The choice of an organized JudeoChrIslamic theology represents that hybrid strategy of survival. Why do we have to choose between the monolithic extremes of a materialist J.D. Barrow or a mystic Feyerabend and his "Tyranny of Science" distorsions?

Observables-based science methodology and metaphysical logic-based epistemology are and will be incomplete as long as there is not a human genetic mutation or a perceptual/ontological reality can exist and be conceptually/epistemologically described or explained in the absence of a human brain.

SUMMARY AND CONCLUSIONS

Neither can an exclusively objective scientific materialism methodology nor an exclusively subjective theological cult can ever formulate a monolithic and unified world view. Neither ideology can articulate the ultimate and absolute structural or functional features of that totality which exists within the reach of sensory or metaphysical detection. If we had have the magic fortune of simultaneously monitoring the <u>atomic clocks</u> on board of the fast speeding <u>Space Shuttle</u> and the synchronized inertial clocks at the slower moving earth bound space station we would have noticed how the latter clocks ran faster on solid earth than those in the accelerating space shuttle! How is that 'time-dilation' **fact** be described and/or explained on the exclusive basis of a scientific observation? Can we dispense of metaphysical explanations based on quantum probabilities and relativity? Not yet. Was that observation an absolute truth? No, because it depends on the objects/events being observed and their respective <u>reference frames</u>. Time will probably show that as the ongoing effort continues on ways to reconcile quantum theory and general relativity dimensional details we will need to expand our poetry to include in a special way additional dreamed dimensions unrelated to either space or time as we have experienced it, a new <u>superspace</u> to accommodate quantum gravity!

Dr. Angell O. de la Sierra, Esq. Deltona, Florida August 15/2012.

7 Is Absolute Introspective Self Knowledge an Illusion?

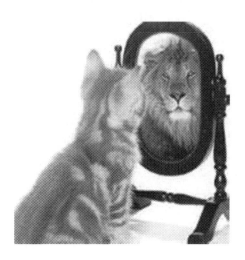

INTRODUCTION

The Spanish philosopher Ortega y Gasset's dictum that humans cannot ever divorce themselves from their ongoing biopsychosocial (BPS) circumstance ("El hombre es el y su circumstancia.") posits one of the most intriguing questions about human behavior when confronted with real-time, relevant existential, ongoing contingencies during the decision-making process. If our human species proudly claim being the protagonists of a neo-Copernican revolution that situates us at the very center of the universe because of being uniquely endowed with the marvel of being able to report on a conscious, introspective journey into ourselves, then it is proper to investigate the expected invariance of that solid knowledge base supporting our decision making activity when confronting and solving contingencies threatening the biopsychosocial equilibrium? The successful evolution of the species depends on the solidity of our self knowledge base. How is a real-time human being going to find that quotidian solution that is both simultaneously relevant, adaptive and at the same time, transcending its immediate immanent character, to become the absolute standard of righteousness independent of any variations in the circumstantial aspects surrounding the specific contingency? From the perspective of a universal standard, can our human species escape his circumstantial shadow that inexorably follows him regardless of his conscious awareness of its possibly negative impact presence? If we were to trust recorded history accounts, only a few individuals successfully resisted the convenience drive of his biopsychosocial circumstance and opted, 'contra natura', to swim against the strong current and altruistically act against self-interest conveniences to set universal standards of behavior for others to emulate in the Ten Commandments Decalon, Tables of the Law, Koran, etc. We call them the historical prophets. What guides them, where is their source of inspiration and guidance, how is righteousness transformed into a living reality? Informed speculations and conjectures are thus in order to at least answer the how, e.g., the BPS sub-model of Reciprocal Transcendental Information Transfer between the human neo cortex and transfinity. At this time we find it necessary to further expand briefly on the nature of the complex question being asked. Are some humans in history 'more special than others connecting with that mysterious 'source' regardless of their preceding formal training in ethics, axiology, etc. To follow, we will try an objective analytical perambulatory dissection of this issue, how do we gain and use knowledge.

ARGUMENTS

One can gain ontological knowledge about the immediate external world and internal body-proper phenomenal environment with the aid of instrumental recordings from external receptors like in vision, audition, taste, touch, temperature, etc. or with internal proprioceptors, stretch receptors, muscle spindles, chemoreceptors, etc. We establish their ontological status by the more reliable direct measurements of their structure/function or the less reliable spoken accounts/reports or explanations of the subjective qualia experienced. Phenomenologically, these real time, ongoing descriptions entail a minimal form of **self-**consciousness for the experiencing subject due to the immediacy of the object or event being witnessed or otherwise experienced. But, even when we are asked, immediately after the occurrence, to give an account of what happened, how do we know that one's particular mental state, beliefs, desires, sensations, etc. did not significantly influence our reply? That particular mental state happens to be our persisting **self**, our personality, our identity as quoted by the classical Greeks as 'Gnoscete Ipsum' or know thyself. But, is an 'objective' ontological description being modified by 'subjective' epistemological explanations controlled by our immediate and ongoing mind state or a persisting mental state? What controls the decision-making process, convenient short term expediency or long term ethical and moral universal considerations? Is our '**self-knowledge**' data base persistent or subject to expedient and convenient modifications? Phrased differently, is the decision-making process controlled by an introspective self knowledge or by the subconscious genetic and memetic reflex networks? It is the role of the subconscious neuro-humoral control network to provide the necessary adjustments responsible for the biopsychosocial (BPS) equilibrium servo controls, those that makes possible for human beings to reflexly respond to familiar situations as recorded in their memory data base. New unfamiliar situations mobilize additional self conscious resources that makes it possible to adapt to the potentially dangerous novelty on the basis of either BPS needs or conveniences, immanent or transcendental aspirations and rarely, altruistic acts against self interests. There is a very important distinction to be made between knowledge acquired through perceptual familiarity and knowledge acquired by conceptual representations, i.e., knowledge we *describe* with some certainty and knowledge we *explain* by way of inferential symbolic or sentential logical representations of both physical and non-physical properties. When we make normative logical decisions about the relevant non-physical, extra sensory invisibilities only when rooted on falsifiable measurable probable facts about objects and/or events, then we speak with Kantian wisdom, a sort of epistemological naturalism or epistemontology. See Kant's Critique of Pure Reason. When the human experience to be communicated resist statistical apprehension by Bayesian logic, we are now in a very different but equally important psychosocial theological manifold which humans individually adopt as their living truths in harmony with their evolving individualized, real time existential circumstance. As we can see, there are many layers in the content of that self knowledge reservoir we tap when making conscious, freely willed decisions. We hope the reader differentiates this time honored, historically recorded, self evident truths from the typical Sartrean existentialism where individuals live and blindly evolve from moment to moment with no normative guidelines to show the righteous way to behave to preserve the viability of the human species. But, the self evident truth is that we, as a species, have evolved in obvious defiance to the also self evident and reliable natural thermodynamic laws of entropy. Why?

Why do some people lead lives exemplifying moral virtues, prudence and courage, benevolence and compassion notwithstanding the many and various temptations to look exclusively after their own ego centered self interests often at the expense of innocent others, like so many currently elected or appointed politicians? Egoism comes in different flavors, psychic, rational or a deadly combination of both when it evolves into a normative rational mindset where the ultimate aim is to unrelently maximize one's **self**-interest at any cost. A veritable intentional psychopathological state of the likes of Hitler, Stalin, Franco, Napoleon and other brilliant historical non-repentant personalities; these are the diametrical opposites of our historical prophets. If these diametrically opposite extremes of behavior the result of natural inherited intelligence and also not the result of a corresponding circumstantial existential reality, what then is the fundamental difference? In the classical 'Summa Contra Gentiles' it is suggested that through 'divine assistance' some chosen individuals are blessed with a direct and immediate grasp of first principles. This reminds us again to ponder on the nature of that divine assistance as being essentially the ability to harmonize the unavoidable, immanent self BPS interests with the transcendental and universal requirements of virtuosity; like Leibniz conceptualization of theology as a human brain centered effort in the 'chosen ones' to create a "science of law". It is almost impossible for us limited human creatures to conceive of an 'assistance', divine or not, lacking an efficient physical cause, however small in dimensions. Therein lies the mesmerizing attraction of an epistemology rooted primarily on functional reality as experienced, e.g., the Kantian 'synthetic a priori propositions'; also somewhat reminiscent of Locke's faith on what material substances and their powers can do outside our capability of ever measuring their dimensions or functions. But we can always write about the explanatory poetry of a belief or just muse on sheer 'cult' nonsense. Being there, done that. After all, why deny it, human certainty is nothing but an epistemic property of human subjects communicating their beliefs with the assistance of all kinds of convenient metaphysical logic and other axiomatic contraptions, however practically useful they may turn out to be! For those of us addicted with the curiosity for the identification of noumenal reality or first principles we have no choice but to rely on the self evident truth that drives our belief-forming activities. Unfortunately the best guide we humans have is what appears to us as counter intuitive, e.g., those non-physical epistemological conceptualizations that become entities able to produce forces that affect physical objects or events. Last but not least, the Darwinian evolution abstraction may be the result of indirect interpretations about observations but it sure as hell makes sense to speculate, if not believe, that species do change in appearance due to what seems to be a natural process that selects and maintains in nature. This may be necessary to explain how species change but may not be sufficient to explain ALL BPS changes experienced inside our quotidian 4d real time existential cage. 'Evolutionary epistemology' is in! We have to live with it until a better epistemological poetry explanation comes into being, especially when analyzing the 'replication' pathway of the selected change. Spontaneously self sustained? If so, we may have to change all of our physics laws that have been so successful in predicting the probability of future events because they **do not** predict a **spontaneous** increase in complexity of structure or function as we corroborate as happening in recorded history. Finally, it is very tempting to assume that acquiring and reporting knowledge about the external environment shouldn't be different when doing the same in respect to ourselves because, if we accept the premise that reality is in our brains, why go elsewhere? But we have to keep looking and continue to write poetry.

SUMMARY AND CONCLUSSIONS

There is no doubt that most of us humans rely blindly on our introspective memory accounts of our respective lives because they seem infallible and seem to account for at least all of our acquired existential knowledge, the rest of our knowledge is in genetic data bases we cannot change at will. After all, it seems odd that we should feel that what we are thinking about in any given moment is not true! Yet, how can we be certain we are capable of attaining a third person perspective about our self attributions free from higher order inferences adopted from prefab 'theories of mind' or behavioral influences? See Dennet. Interestingly we have analyzed (see articles on intra and interspecies information transfer) how we may be utilizing same brain circuitry, especially mirror neurons, in gaining reliable insights about our own mental states as we do in others. In this simulation effort we may learn of other's states of mind by using their facial expression cues in a given situation and then projecting oneself empathically into the other's situation, i.e., allowing the observer through a special mode of self-reflection, to experience what one would believe or desire, feel, etc. if we were in that situation oneself. We had hoped to use similar arguments to explain how the use of similar brain processing circuitry may be activated when receiving information from transfinity sources, if any. We have argued that this 'simulation theory certainty' needs to be qualified and improved on.

When we are asked to report on our personal account of, e.g., an accident we had just witnessed, how many persons may '**consciously**' report relevant objects, events or sensations 'experienced' but **not** strictly present inside our perceptual field or emotional mindset during the occurrence? Was it influenced by the reporter's current and ongoing mindset or was it objective even when it would carry negative consequences to the reporter or to his special others? Why the inconsistency? Is this the result of the inevitable **subconscious** influence from individualized circumstances, e.g., sensations, emotions, appetites, etc. or was it always the result of a **conscious** deliberate intention to benefit from the consequences? Are we really having those thoughts and sensations reported, are they true? There is no unanimous consensus as to how to evaluate the results of introspective reports, or what weight to accord 'other sources'. Introspection therefore faces an especially complex problem of standard of calibration. Should we rely on what often seems to be an exalted epistemic claim made on behalf of introspective self consciousness as being true and very distinct from the brain epistemic processing we use in other domains, i.e., on what credible basis can we claim that there is a fundamental difference between self-knowledge and other-knowledge? What is obviously distinct is the leisurely, scholarly addictive habit of the few retired to indulge in poetry writing about the complexities of self and the many others sharing the same ecological niche, very different from the quotidian existential reality of the surviving, unemployed and stressed many others coexisting with us. Nothing wrong with writing poetry so long as you keep your feet on the solid grounds of real time existence as you look at the stars for guidance and then take the first step 'ad astra per asperas'.

Dr. Angell O. de la Sierra, Esq. Deltona, Florida Summer 2012

 Quo Vadis Evolution? The Immanent 'Invariant' and the Transcendental Transforming Horizons

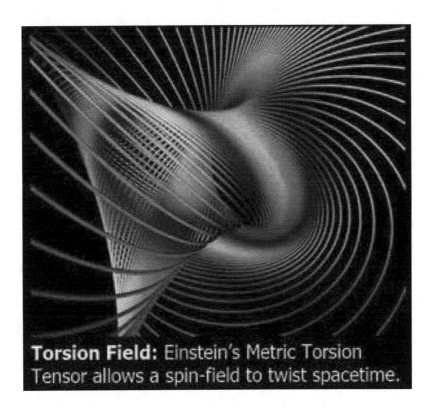

Torsion Field: Einstein's Metric Torsion Tensor allows a spin-field to twist spacetime.

INTRODUCTION

At some point in our lives we all have experienced and enjoyed the immense pleasure of anintrospective, self conscious trip into ourselves, a kind of self-induced solitary confinement from the surrounding crowds, trying to ponder on the physically invariant aspects of our individualized existential reality, the **what** of 'I' vis a vis 'the other', i.e., trying to explain to yourself why some things do change while others apparently remain the same, wondering **how** you got where you are and **where** will you go, if anywhere, **when** you . . . . and everyone else die, quo vadis? More often than not you feel overwhelmed by the super complexity of the physical sensory phenomena reaching consciousness, not to mention the equally experienced qualia originating from the extrasensory/metaphysical object or event invisible to our direct sensory detection or measurement. Then, in frustration, you conclude that 'the more things change, the more they remain the same', "vivir es ver volver" (life is to see same things past come back)? But, if you are afflicted by the 'sane psychosis' of curiosity, then you make it a hobby to meditate deep about the **why,** using whatever information resources, whatever science, technology and metaphysical logic has been placed within your reach. But the conclusions are disappointing when we find out that other subhuman species enjoy lower thresholds to the same sensory information and we discover that our human brain natural combinatorial capacity without the aid of instruments is dismally low. Yet, we all witness the self-evident truths about the Newtonian apple falling to the ground, rain water streaming down hill, the loss of structure and/or function of complex objects falling from high buildings or contrariwise, the required supply of externally applied energy or effort to make same object move or spontaneously restructure itself when returning to its original locus in the tall building. A closer look will immediately evidence that complexly structured objects or events exhibit either a bilateral or rotational symmetry, the kind of ordered complexity that was never the result of natural spontaneous processes. On the other hand, the loss of order and complexity, as when a tall building naturally collapses, brings all systems to a minimum of free energy and a corresponding increase in entropy. Then we observe, with Pierre Curie, that the symmetry elements of the causes must be found in their effects while the converse is not true, i.e., the effects can be more symmetric than the causes.

Is evolution fueled by asymmetry, induced by external forces or spontaneous? Then we wonder like Leibniz did in his 'Principle of Sufficient Reason' (PSR): Why so?

Then we also naturally posit the intervention of an efficient causal agency as the driving force behind this transformational change in the direction of a lesser entropy content (negentropy) and increased organizational complexity. If there is no **sufficient reason** for one thing to happen instead of another, the Leibniz principle says that nothing will happen and the initial situation will not change. What then is the efficient causal agency in defiance of natural laws and why? Where in infinity or transfinity is this agency located? Maybe inside our own human brains? If the latter, since it cannot spontaneously come into being, where—if anywhere—is the external source of inspirational righteousness originating the information being transferred to our decisional human brain lobe? The simplest way to start digging into this analysis is to postpone the identification of the source and start with the relatively easier chore of characterizing the kind of information being transferred . . . . or settle for the complex structural/functional evolutionary changes resulting therefrom? To differentiate the constituent elements of complexity we notice, prima facie, order in structure and function of either single sensory objects or in situations where interacting sensory objects describe a measurable event. This is the proper domain of the 4-d ontological aspect of the scientific methodology. But much beyond the reaches of this Minkowsky spatio—temporal domain we find the equally relevant epistemological n-1 d metaphysical logic to assist in the explanation of that experienced force which cannot be described experimentally as a physical object or observable event. To follow is a brief exposition of the need for a hybrid epistemontological approach when analyzing existential reality where symmetry considerations play a decisive role in the human brain when processing the information input when ordering the complexities of physical and metaphysical reality.

ARGUMENTATION

We notice that most sensory objects have in common a given symmetry, either a bilateral symmetry (e.g., two arms of a human body statue in anatomical position) or a rotational symmetry (e.g., spherical objects) where there is complete equivalence between the existing alternatives (the left hand with respect to the right hand or a full 360 degree axial rotation of a human statue/spherical object, respectively). As in nature, we also notice that, in the absence of an asymmetric transforming cause (externally applied or self-induced force?), the initial invariant state symmetry is preserved, i.e., a breaking of the original symmetry— whether human-induced or in its highest natural entropy state—cannot happen without a reason because *an asymmetry cannot originate spontaneously.* How then was microscopic and cosmological order 'created'? A tall order for the scientific community to handle with its methodology, imagine now the level of complexity faced when you consider the invariance under a specified group of transformations and the symmetry concept is now applied not only to ontological spatial statues or spherical objects but also to relevant epistemologically abstract virtual 'objects' such as found in metaphysical logic math expressions, e.g., dynamical equations of state.

But the curious mind has to start from the sense-phenomenal physically obvious to the statistically probable, metaphysically inferred and then the theosophically possible explanations model when the effort has exceeded the human brain capacities to epistemontologically hybridize and harmonize all the different elements in the first two as a coherent unit or unitary whole. An extraordinary task when you have to consider the constitutive elements in a single human being made up of trillions of microscopic living cells, the majority of which of different species and each, not only following their individualized trajectories through the Many World universes according to the idiosyncrasies of their many molecules, atoms, subatomic particles, etc., but also tracking the evolutionary path of the unit human life to its ultimate destination. Yet you are able to maintain through life the 'singularity' of your unit body and mind as it invariantly persist while changing. In other words, you are simultaneously a statistically invariant, physico-chemical **you** and a constantly transforming **many**, while you traverse a world line in one or many universes . . . . going somewhere.

So, historically we start by a classification of sensory reality according to their varied symmetry, structural macro properties as manifested in harmony, beauty, and unity followed by their inferred micro structural properties after their epistemological translation into irreducible representations of their fundamental physical symmetry groups, e.g., a group-theoretical account of objects or their canonical Hamiltonian representation as dynamic entities. The next step was to harmonize the invariant geometrical abstractions with the dynamic Hamiltonian equations of motion. The complex evolving dynamic theories of nature were made easier to comprehend by Jacobi with the strategy of applying transformations of the dynamic variables that leave the Hamiltonian equations invariant. This way the original formulation became thereby transformed into a new one that is simpler but perfectly equivalent albeit somewhat removed from the existential reality it purports to substitute for. May this be carrying symmetry principles too far, the reason why general relativity and quantum physics cannot be integrated into a unit theory and allow both to reconcile. We briefly analyzed this constrain in a previous chapter.

From both an *ontological* and epistemological perspective, symmetries in theories represent properties existing in nature that characterize the structure and function of the physical world as illustrated by their methodological success in predicting the existence of new particles in physics, e.g., the prediction of the W and Z particles in the unification of the weak and electromagnetic interactions. Of course some symmetries are observed while others are only inferred and thus validated by their predictive value. It would seem as if symmetries represent natural, minimum free energy states in equilibrium. As such they serve the purpose of being used as constraints on the evolution of new physical theories, a valuable normative role assuring the compatibility of quantities, dimensions and form in their constitutive equations.

This is especially important now while we struggle to find a unified description of all the fundamental forces of nature (gravitational, weak, electromagnetic and strong) in terms of underlying local symmetry groups. Hopefully the unification is just as credible at the explicit, measurable, ontological level as it may be at the implicit representational/epistemological levels, i.e., observably invariant global space time symmetry and the inferred locally varying continuous symmetry. In our opinion all symmetry principles are operational transcendental strategies aimed at making our understanding of the world more intelligible with no guarantee of reaching reality 'in se'. But, there is indeed a natural connection between the invariables and structural realism just like between symmetry and *objectivity*, the validity of which is predicated on being the same for all observers and do not depend on any particular perspective under which is being considered. Objective realism is that which remains invariant no matter how many transformations it suffered when forced into a convenient reference frame. Can we make the same claim for what seems the human-contrived epistemological explanations of transfinite dynamic invisibilities 'existing' beyond the human 4-d spatiotemporal Minkowsky cage?

Why did the human species historically and conveniently choose the invariant features of symmetry to explain his dynamic evolution through space time? Was it unconsciously genetically/biologically determined, subconsciously mimetically/psychosocially imposed by circumstantial/environmental constraints or is it the inevitable consequence of the freely willed, self conscious effort of a few historical prophets inspired by transfinite 'revelations' guiding their efforts through the pathways of righteousness to preserve life, psychic comfort and social conviviality, i.e., create and sustain a biopsychosocial (BPS) equilibrium through life?

The common denominator found in a BPS equilibrium is 'symmetry', whether discovered or invented in the mathematical proportions and harmonies they contain, or the related properties and beauty of their form. A combination of an essential biological, life preserving effort and the convenience of a happy psychosocial environment in guarantee of the survival of human life and self consciousness. The symmetric proportions of material objects not only have an esthetic appeal (beauty, regularity and unity) but, when deliberately designed by the architect or engineer as e.g., the regular polygons, polyhedrals, etc. as the structural foundations of buildings, factories, etc., the geometry is defined in terms of their invariance under specified groups of rotations and reflections, not necessarily esthetic criteria. No wonder the current appeal of differential geometry and topology to theoretical physicists when explaining the invisible domain of relevant sub atomic and cosmological reality. This time symmetry considerations propitiated the development of group-theoretic representations that have been so useful in modern physics to create 'equivalent groups' by symmetry transformations easier to exchange with one another without allegedly substantially changing the unit wholeness being considered. In our opinion, this may introduce non-compatible elements into general formulations affecting their claimed invariance under the transformation when equivalent elements are exchanged according to one of the specified mathematical operations, as the case may be. Having perhaps reached the limits of human instrumental resolution in the description of objects or phenomena, we have now emphasized more the application of *symmetry principles* to natural laws in our attempt to achieve a *unity of different and equal elements* in our explanations/conceptualizations of reality which has become central to modern physics. There are always serious problems when you hybridize invariant symmetry principles with transforming symmetry arguments into a unit whole theory.

SUMMARY AND CONCLUSIONS

Needless to say, the professions of medicine, law and engineering practitioners have been more efficient in doing their 'thing' than their academic philosophy equivalents in the same areas because the former are mostly dealing with the ontologically and statistically invariant macro aspects of 4-d space time reality while the latter must conceptually keep simultaneous control of both invariant and transforming aspects of real time existential and virtual universal models of the same reality. The application of symmetry principles has provided ontology and epistemology useful tools to discover the structure and function of absolute reality, all within the known perceptual and conceptual limitations of the human observer to find/identify noumenal reality.

The most successful efforts in that direction have been to control the dynamic Hamiltonian formulations of measurable phenomena by conveniently holding them as invariant by the use of transforming operations of the relevant variables in the dynamic equations (Jacobian transforms). This way the intractable dynamics are transformed into simpler but perfectly equivalent now amenable to to combine, permute, exchange with equivalent representations, etc. Whether this simplification correspond to reality, quare!

We have dramatized the complexity of reality by reminding the reader that the historical, lifetime chronology of a single living human being is a macro statistical description conveniently ignoring the concomitant evolutionary path of trillions of microscopic living entities, mostly of different subhuman species, e.g., bacteria, molds, etc., each cell, molecule, atom, subatomic particle, etc following independent trajectories through the various Multiverse options. Yet the unitary integrity of your physical body and mental idiosyncrasies remain distinguishable whether you traverse a world line in one universe, or many.

Because of the successful influence of symmetry principles in scientific methodology pursuits, as outlined above, we do not appreciate as much its impact on the metaphysical logic of our explanatory models of existential and abstract/virtual reality equivalents. We briefly discussed two outstanding influences, the Leibnizean Principle of Sufficient Reason (PSR) and Pierre Curie's theory of causality. PSR stresses the correlation between symmetry (bilateral or rotational) and natural stability implied in the complete equivalence between the existing alternatives, as discussed above, e.g., if the alternative positions are equivalent why choose among them (invariance). This means that in the absence of an asymmetric efficient cause there is no reason to change, i.e., a breaking of the initial symmetry cannot happen without a reason, or *an asymmetry cannot originate spontaneously* without defying laws of nature, yet it happens, as argued.

In a related argument, Pierre Curie, argues that the symmetry elements of the causes must be found in their effects while the converse is not true, i.e., the effects can be more symmetric than the causes. And we ask: is evolution fueled by asymmetry, induced by external forces or spontaneous?

As a parting 'lei motif' coda allow me to philosophize a little on what I have tried to market in the previous chapters of these volumes: "The Hypothetical 'How' Integrating the What, Where, When, Who and Why of the Constitutive Elements of 4-d Human Existential Reality."

This brief exposition could have been entitled "Reciprocal Information transfer between human species and n-dimensional space.", or "From here to eternity and back." for that matter. It naturally follows from my two previous chapters on 'intraspecies' and 'interspecies' information transfer respectively. Within the contextual guidelines of the 'epistemontological hybrid, biopsychosocial (BPS) model, the 'what' refers to the information content (matter, energy) whether ontologically *described* in its intraspecies transition from sensory receptors to consciousness or epistemologically *explained* as it reciprocally travels to and from an n-dimensional space. The rest is my sheer wishful thinking poetry. The expressions are ontologically rooted on *observables* from the scientific methodology arsenal and on epistemological inferences from metaphysical logic axioms/tautologies where reduction to symbolic or sentential logic representations has been deliberately reduced here to a minimum to reach all informed audiences. The 'epistemontological' hybrid approach will become obvious if we can imagine the linear temporal transition of either a visible sphere or a line in our real-time Minkosky 4-d macro space as these structures sequentially halve their dimension until they escape unaided sensory or instrumental detection (from magnifying glass to electron microscopy). As the *described* features of 'what' enter an invisible extrasensory domain we have no reason to believe it has existentially disappeared (as long as we 'sense' its relevant effects) simply because we may have to resort now to *explanations* as to its probable presence somewhere in space. While it may originally sound counterintuitive, it is not difficult to imagine, e.g., the basketball size becoming a softball size, a tennis ball, a ping-pong ball, a marble size, etc. until it eventually becomes a zero dimensional point singularity, invisible to us because it has transcended/escaped our sense detection inside our 4-d sense-phenomenal state. Same argument applies to the visible line—or any other geometry imaginable—transition towards a spherical point singularity. Likewise we can imagine a not so linear, stepwise and reversible sequential flow of information projecting from different geometries inside or outside our sensory sphere of detection (which we conveniently may represent as 3 dimensions of space xyz and one of time) to form our 4-d Minkowsky sensory world. We can either choose 3 lines diverging from same origin 'o' at right angles to each other or use spherical coordinates inside a geodesic. This reverse flow of information arriving eventually to a particular receptor as a zero-dimensional quantum energy unit sphere (wave) to and fro all of space or hyperspace, whether relevant or not to the human species quotidian experience carries important information to our environment. Upon arrival it will release its energy content on any particle, atom, molecular, cellular, tissue, organ or macrostructure containing/vibrating at the appropriate phase and resonant frequency energy that makes coupling/entanglement and transmission of information possible, e.g., an incomplete electron orbit in a vibrating atom/molecule inside a DNA spiral, photosynthetic chromophores or wiggling protein string receptors. At the brain level this entanglement or collapse of the wave function with all appropriate receptor configurations provides the background noise waves we described earlier in the EEG responsible for amplification of subthreshold energy transfer (intra and interspecies) from the internal/external environment.

There are many—obvious and not so obvious—geometrical reasons why information (matter/energy, particle/wave) should travel optimally as spherical quanta but we find it mathematically convenient to represent their transient location using spherical coordinates or inside a 3-d (xyz) cubical space to be able to answer the 'where' question about the spatio-temporal position of the 'what' wave/particle (wavicle) in a given moment in time either inside or outside our sensory/visible or extrasensory/invisible domain or manifold.

Notice that any geometry, e.g., polygon, is a sphere in potency as it sequentially diminishes its size, as discussed.

If we stretch our imagination it should not be difficult to visualize that, as the pure energy content E diminishes in the smallest spherical massless quantum, a particle M will be created from the condensate according to the correlation between mass and energy given by E= MC2. A dimensionless sphere singularity 'a' has unit 'matter'/information moving to and fro across space and hyperspace until detected or otherwise captured by an appropriate resonant receptor, visual, olfactory, audible or otherwise.

Consider now how, in locating 'a''s matter/energy ('what') photon singularity's position in space, we can also increase its information content and, from an assumed linear trajectory, identify a second point 'b' along its path at variable distances from its origin 'o'. The resulting *line* can now provide information about positions (its own/another object) along such 'ab' line as it extends into or returns from n-d space by developing a uni-dimensional linear algebra. By adding a third point 'c' outside line ab we create a 2-d plane and, by measuring the angle sustained as the line rotates from the origin 'o' (e.g., at 'a' or 'b') to reach the third point 'c'. Now we are creating a vector calculus to explain the position of a wavicle in both the previous 2-d plane or the new 3-d world scenario more consistent with our sense-phenomenal reality experience. Now we continue to add information on 'where' by indicating how far and in what direction either point 'c' or any other object along the line crossing line 'oc' as it extends into or returns from n-d space—whether inside the 3-d sensory box/geodesic or beyond.

Notice also that this way, yet another visible or invisible point/object 'd' need not be either on the 2-d xy plane created (embedded above or below it) or along the oà'c' line to be identified. If so, by extending a line from 'o' to 'c' we have created a third dimension z, improving on our ability to describe any point/object 'd' location *anywhere* inside new 3-d space created or in hyperspace (as long as being possibly detected along line 'od', unless another 3-d/ geodesic is subsequently created with point 'd' as the new origin), i.e., this way we can create additional location units in space and hyperspace as long as the complexity of the required analytical algebras and computing resources do not get unwieldy, e.g., by extending a line from 'c' → 'd', 'd' → 'e', etc.

Depending on the object/point distance from the original reference point 'o' we can develop the algebras describing the time unit increments to get from point to point or line to line, sphere to sphere, etc. and, by describing how fast ('t') an object covers that distance D, we invent the concepts of Velocity = dD/t and acceleration = dV/dt and thereby increase the information content on the 'where' is the matter/energy 'what' is coming from or going to and incorporating it in our concept of a 4-d spatiotemporal unit sphere a la Minkowsky.

Having accepted the convenience of this unit of localization 'where' we are also describing the 'when' as the time element gets incorporated into the 3-d space dimension. Of course the 'what' need not be sitting static waiting to be identified, it can be dynamically spinning on an axis, rotating with precessional movements, revolving, etc. where each change in the position of a given point requires the appropriate analytical construction of the suggested 4-d or geodesic unit. To illustrate, in a 4-d space, a vector displays a particular behavior when acted upon by a rotation or when reflected in a plane surface. Such spatial rotations and reflections provide additional information about the causal dynamics and are best expressed in differential geometry representations using Lie or Clifford algebras to describe the complex geometry in terms of spinors (Seeorientationentanglement at http://en.wikipedia.org/wiki/Orientation_entanglement).

It should be noticed that the implication of a trajectory of unit matter/energy is linear along the straight lines joining 2 points or restricted to lines lying on the 2 surfaces of planes formed by joining 3 points or the interior/exterior surfaces or inside the interior volumes of the 3d structures formed when leaving the 2-d plane surface. We know that measured experimental trajectories, e.g., along the surface area of a 2-d plane, may show maxima/minima variations along a 1-d line (on the plane) before reaching its destination, e.g., recursive cycles that when moving along a straight line appear as sine waves in a Fourier analysis, etc., and that these trajectories vary according to the influence of other *adjacent* locations along its path.

Yet, it should not be difficult to see the convenience of representing any point/object location *anywhere* in n-d space as a localized 4-d Minkowsky space using spherical coordinates for analytical purposes. The task is being able to trace the path of its origin and/or destiny. After all a spherical adimensional point singularity represents the hypothetical origin/end of a reversible transmission of matter/energy wavicles between 2 locations anywhere in n-d space which can evolve from a massless energy source into an integrated traveling, invisible wavicle in hyperspace or the visible object inside our sensory 4-d space by the accretion of coincident points entangling by resonant phase coupling or otherwise, i.e., any multidimensional object or adimensional singularity can transmit its constitutive information (mass/energy content) by differentiation/integration into simpler/complex units of transfer approaching as a limit the unit spherical quantum configuration or the observable object as the case may be. This way, the visible transmitter differentiates into quantum spherical units for projections traveling at speeds exceeding the speed of light into new locations inside sensory 4-d space and beyond while the receiver receptor(s) integrate(s) the information units into new visible objects in space or hyperspace by resonant phase coupling entanglement.

The most fascinating result of this model of matter/energy information transfer is that it allows for an analysis/understanding of a few other counterintuitive albeit self-evident observable facts in apparent violation of natural laws as will briefly be expanded below, e.g., negentropy as seen in the synthesis of order out of disorder when making conscious free will decisions. The reversible energy/mass information transfer to and fro between a source and its receptor destination seems to be characterized as being a quantum/discontinued, non-linear, non local, asymmetric but **not necessarily** an energy dissipating entropic event as witnessed by self-evident sense-phenomenal and historical manifestations, e.g., spontaneous and self-sustained cosmic/institutional order and life generation. Hence the paradox of two co-existing systems, a visible deterministic *described* by the scientific methodology and an invisible indeterministic *explained* by metaphysic logic; a probable world, held indelibly together by the probabilities of quantum theory provisions—in a hybrid indelible epistemontological unit. This cognitive approach makes possible a different view of existential reality as an equilibrium between the biological, psychic and social survival imperatives tailored to individualized complex circumstantial factors in the biosphere niche.

In the process it opens the doors ajar for further explorations on the possibility of modeling a new physics to explain the mesoscopic quantum world by integrating the input contributions originating from many vital body sources (neuro-endocrine, immune, genetic, etc.) and/or n-d space. This would be the result of viewing the reversible transition between the micro subplanckian level and the macro cosmological n-d level via the visible 4-d mesoscopic level as resulting from the integration of invisible Planck constant quantum units of matter/energy and/or volumes as they reach or leave macro quantum phases to reach visible levels of identification using same mathematical transfer strategies as discussed. This possibility comes as the result of analyzing the information/energy transfer across domains/manifolds as discussed under quantum transfer of Planck units (constants) and now viewed as the possibility of dealing in addition with massive but invisible dark matter in our midst. This view is made possible when we briefly examine further what was explained above about the new manifolds appearing as we transcend (symmetry breaking) the 4-d space constraints into micro or macro hyperspace. Some have characterized these adjacent levels as onion peels, layered sheaths, Bohr orbitals, etc. of space-time units. Could the convergence of these many massless unit singularities (or biophoton aggregates thereof) on brain matter constitute the invisible supercomplex mind state? Quare.

Our quotidian existential reality, as experienced in the ecosystem niche of our biosphere, gets individually configured inside an ordinary 4-d space-time sensory reality and the attending biopsychosocial circumstances as described mostly by the natural sciences. Yet we know there is more to it than meets the eye that influences our decision-making process, especially our psychic and social behavior details . . . things that defy rationality and common sense at times. Well, it so happens that we find similar conclusions stemming from the results we see when playing around with mathematical logic, things like imaginary lines going back to infinity, non locality, a particle being in 2 different locations simultaneously, etc.

What we must remember is that our human species has limited capacity for the sensory resolution of 'real' objects/events even inside our ordinary 4-d space, not to mention the limitations in brain combinatorial capacity to analyze variables exceeding a limited number of objects or events even though their shape/form or location are invisible they somehow may substantially influence our daily lives. Enter metaphysics to complete the reality picture.

The strictly human features allowing these cognitive incursions into the invisible domains are our ability for introspective search for self and our language ability to describe how we differ from others as expressed/represented in logic symbols or sentences. Man is back at the center of the universe, a neo-Copernican revolution?

First we observe that an infinite regression in size of any geometrical 3-d structure comes to a spherical point, visible in our unaided 4-d reality or not. Then we realize that in the reverse sequence material geometries probably started with a point also, visible or not! We have tentatively 'discovered' 'how' the essence of the 'what' has ontological descriptions and epistemological explanatory inferences about their presence, especially when outside the sensory 4-d reality. Then we form a line by joining 2 points and we discover 'how' we can represent the probable location ('where') of that invisible point if located along the 1-d extension of the line 'from here to eternity'. If outside that line, I form another line by joining 3 points to form a 2-d plane surface where it may be located along any line contained inside (above or below) the 2 surfaces formed. As mentioned above, we can develop a vector calculus to locate any point on the plane by, e.g., measuring the angular displacement of 2 intersecting lines with a common origin. We can develop a plane geometry to improve on the localization ('where') of any point ('what') in that surface, e.g., Euclidean geometry, Pythagoras theorem, etc. We have improved our localization of matter/energy from a line 'scalar' to a ''vector'' field. Now an unexpected result surfaces as we discover that, from the innocent $x2+y2=c2$ relationship between the triangular intersecting lines at right angle formed by the 3 points, we discover not only the geometric functions (sine, cosine, etc.) when the plane is a circle but the counterintuitive notions of infinity, recursive cycles, negative numbers, imaginary and complex numbers, etc., all by manipulating the symbolic representations! However, an object in a vector field can change strength and direction when acting as a source or can experience them as a destination, e.g., a migratory bird in flight under the effects of earth's gravitational field when the strength and distance of the field varies as a function of time.

If we now want to locate a point 'z' located **outside** the plane (above or below) we extend a line from a point origin on the xy plane to z creating in the process a 3-d cubical unit space or unit sphere (geodesical) as explained in solid and space geometries thus creating our unit 4-d space that enables us to trace and thus *explain* the probable origin/destination or location of matter/energy sources or destinations of at least unit spherical singularities which can be further geometrically embellished to accommodate other degrees of freedom emerging in their trajectory and resulting from internal/external influences, e.g., tensor and spinor fields that better explains the dynamics of forces acting at a distance and hoping to better explain the phenomenon of cosmological 'non-locality' of the Einstenian 'spooky actions at a distance'.

When the bird flies in a straight line scalar the vector becomes a 0-order tensor but when other influences (describable also as vectors) come into play, the order of the tensor increases depending on the number of participating vectors in a given space-time location. Any number of the 5 known forces in nature (gravity, electricity, magnetism, etc.) and their strength at a given point in space-time (when explained as vectors) are then represented as the elements of a particular matrix for analytical and evaluation purposes without defining the type/nature of influence being considered, gravitational or otherwise. It is important to realize that each participating force creates its own time-line that can either coincide or intersect others and thus creating thereby 3 additional dimensions of time for a 6-d hyperspace, without including other time-lines generated by other rotational forces present (spin, precession, wobbling, etc.) all possibly being integrated in our BPS model into a resultant 'existential' location inside an expanded, real-time unit 4-d space.

So much for this brief orientation on the probable location ('where') of the matter/energy ('what') participating in the dynamic synthesis/degradation at a given moment in time ('when') of that 4-d sense-phenomenal view we refer to as our human existential reality. But the unit 4-d sphere concatenation of n-d locations model cannot now, if ever, explain/ identify the force behind the reversible flow of energy/matter between us and others across n-d space, the 'who' and 'why' of existential reality. These answers we leave to poets and theologians who provide evolving transitory palliatives to substitute for the unreachable and invisible Omega point(s) at either infinite 'end' of the reversible flow along the dis-continuum path. The easy answer is to dismiss it as, "it's all in your head". No brain, no reality, no consciousness.

Maybe for us pitiful humans, life is not about having arrived but about getting there as we travel along an asymptotic path . . . A long time ago I was impressed when I observed in my biophysics lab at Sloan Kettering Institute in New York the sequential transformation of elongated chick embryo fibroblasts grown in cultures to spherical invasive cancer cells by just adding a white powder (Rous Sarcoma virus) from a test tube to the Petri Dish! I was determined to explain how an inanimate ribonucleotide molecule can be animated to invade and infect and transform other normal cells as observed with the electron microscope. Rubin and Temin modeled what I couldn't see and won them a Nobel prize, the ribonucleotide virus had become associated with the host's DNA! Later on I was again perplexed to record brain activity from implanted electrodes in a hungry cat's reticular mesencephalic area isolated from any possibility of sensory input (blinded, in a positive pressure cage in a closed room). This happened when either food or another cat from the opposite sex approached from afar! In another setting, I was able to call the attention of a lady sitting in front of me during a conference, almost at will. I couldn't wait to retire and work on these spooky experiences.

Years of study and three volumes on "Neurophilosophy of Consciousness" published later I still have not been able to explain, let alone describe, the identity of the 'who' if any or the mysterious 'why'. One often wonders what would be the result of an experimental paradigm shift emphasizing on man as the center and reason for all things existing, in the visible sense-phenomenal 4-d and the invisible, extrasensory n-d domains. Perhaps if we become committed to spend (or waste) time studying/exploring those intangible imaginary numbers, non-local actions at a distance, negative time, simultaneous presence of one particle in two locations, information transfer at the speed of light, dark matter and other invisibilities we will move closer to Omega along the asymptotic line . . . For starters, concentrate on the mesoscopic level and trace the conceptual path of an invisible Planck's energy quantum singularity as it builds up by accretion into the sense reality of the mesoscopic level where dark matter considerations will probably show its need of inclusion. It may not be far-fetched that the probable explanation of the unit 4-d existential reality will be formulated in terms of scaled-up/scaled-down subsets of unit mass/energy quantum content reversibly traveling to and fro the extreme ends of micro and cosmic reality as the dark/fractal hierarchies become distinguishable/detected inside our existential, sense-phenomenal 4-d mesoscopic reality.

EPILOGUE

This Volume V (Neurophilosophy of Consciousness) is a continuation of the previous volume that did not make it into press on time and represents an update on the status of consciousness as viewed within the context of an evolving perspective of human brain dynamics as evidenced by both modern technologies and new mathematical abstractions. One thing has been clear to this author, yes this is a 'Brave New World' worth discovering but we are shifting our emphasis too much into the vagaries of metaphysical abstractions at the expense of losing the ontological perspective of that evolving brain dynamics that makes it possible. It would seem as if our new physical materialist theoretical physicists and philosophers prefer to ignore that historical revolution that put man and his ongoing existential circumstances back at the center of the universe, like Husserl's phenomenology, e.g., Heidegger's *existentiale Analytik*, Ortega y Gasset's 'perspectivism', Dilthey's Leben philosophie and others. It is like ignoring that it was a human brain existing in a continuously evolving dynamic process of self transformation continues to un-relentlessly modify and reformulate his understanding of life experiences, rejecting the notion that if it was valid for the preceding 'classic' generation it is still viable in the modern convulsive 21th.century today. The work of these 'existentialists' was mostly based on the lessons learned from recorded history but, important as it is as a source, we have to remember that history is a synthesis of facts where psychosocial circumstances heavily influenced human motives, behaviors and retaliations, i.e., historical facts are not necessarily objectively based on falsifiable facts in evidence. Likewise, the laws of nature are not necessarily always determined by the same particles interacting under similar circumstances. These two extreme positions need a contemporaneous update before they are reconciled and ultimately hybridized into a coherent epistemontological whole. Neither should we accept the supremacy of the general, abstracts conceptualizations endorsed by materialist physics nor its total rejection as 'irrelevant' by radical empiricists that rather opt for the Sartrean type of day in and day out hedonistic existentialism. The temporality of evolutionary phenomenological and metaphysical logic change is very much part of reality. Natural cycles seem to repeat in cycles but only in appearance because the complete cycle was more of a spiral than a circle of repetition. As discussed *below in the Einstenian-Bohr debate on the reality of the simultaneous verification of a particle's position and momentum, the verifiable 'here and now' is as important as the hypothesized predictable 'later', one reality but at different times, the verifiable present is best understood than an unverifiable conceptualization, albeit predictable (always?). In our BPS model we welcome the verifiable measurement or observation along with the transcendental reduction (Husserl's abstract analogical transposition) as the best compromise for a fundamental basis in the understanding the experience of reality

The logic behind this epistemontological approach is simple, the human existential reality experienced is an individualized elaboration of the brain determined by genetic, learned and undefined yet other possible influences that theosophical credo thrive on in their modeling of biopsychosocial, ergo human life is the ultimate reality. Consequently the biopsychosocial equilibrium with circumstantial conditions that we share with the subhuman living beings is necessary for day to day survival but not sufficient to guarantee the human species survival across generations. Unfortunately that guarantee is predicated on an efficient functional formulation of that relevant, falsifiable reality outside perceptual and/or conceptual threshold. It is not enough to exclusively study the details of human biopsycho social equilibrium (Ortega's metaphysics of the 'elan vital'), but neither is the exclusive abstract reduction to symbolic formulation of invisibilities, relevant or not, like extreme radical religionists do, theosophies and materialist physicists alike. Human need not become neither the willing prisoners of the theoretical physicists' objectivism nor the biological research scientist objectivism to feed the ego or other self serving interests of their intellectual proponents because existence is inexorably about **both** real perspectives, no principle can be superior to life . . . , all lives. To quote Ortega y Gasset: ". . . , "my life"—in the "biographical" not in the "biological" sense—is the question of what to do with it and that of what happens to me as I find myself "shipwrecked" in the precarious sea of "circumstances."

For unknown reasons beyond my capacities to analyze, our human species has been uniquely endowed with the means to survive thanks to his introspective ability to ". . . sink into the inner depths of his being as he or she makes an effort to hold on to consciousness and to the very essence of his life . . . . (because) "To live," . . . "is to deal with the world, aim at it, act in it, be occupied with" (*Obras*, 5: 26, 33-34, 35, 44-45, 7: 103-04, Ortega). As we argue, the experience of existential living is not about some scientific description of fMRI brain recordings or some metaphysical logic principle underlying such observations unless the real life historical and psychosocial dimensions are incorporated into the equation.

For those respectful colleagues of mine in academia who keep insisting that my strategy all along—based on my publications—has consisted on deliberately or subconsciously marketing a Roman Catholic cosmogony without calling it by name, I rest on the literal interpretation of my writings by others in the general public. Like everyone else, we all have preferences that may be relevant or not to a particular domain of discourse. If nothing else it proves my point about judgments based on other than factual data as briefly mentioned below in relation to quantum non-locality. We all have beliefs that are based on individualized circumstances surrounding our cultural upbringing and adult life. That diagnosis on my 'hidden agenda' certainly is not based on signs and symptoms consistently observed or measured because one can be objective in recognizing meaningful content in those opposed to one's views. There existed many good human beings much before organized religions were established.

In any event we hope to have confused readers as much as we still remain ourselves about what the universal guiding principle should be as circumstances evolve into the future. What is or should be the ultimate criterion of truth for the faithful in the JudeoChrIslamic or physical materialist religions? We can also respect the Buddhist conviction that ultimately reality transcends all possible human elaborations and cannot ever be fully comprehended by sensory descriptions or linguistic and conceptual explanation, i.e., it escapes the grasp of language and thoughts representations for analysis. However, while we recognize the human brain sensory and conceptual limitations, it seems unwarranted to conclude that physical objects do not phenomenologically exist or emerge from non-physical empty vacuums.

Another issue worthwhile pointing out in this dilemma of 'which reality is true', if either one. The answer is related to the required reconciliation between quantum theory and general relativity. As we interpret it, the 'criterion of reality' seems to be related to the EPR and Bell's theorem interpretations (based on Bohm's spin measurements) of the **physical** real-time immanent 'locality' (as measured in the lab) and the hoped-for **metaphysical** universality of an alleged 'non-locality', the classical syndrome of confusing the reality of the conceptually inferred map with the reality of the phenomenologically perceptual territory. If we could only simultaneously **measure** or at least predict **both** the evolving and interacting variables then they can be regarded as simultaneous elements of physical reality, seen or unseen. But this is not yet the case for our limited human brain performance, which reality is true?

For the benefit of those more familiar with theoretical physics, the Einstein-Podolsky-Rosen 'solution' constituted an attempt of reconciliation of the phenomenological with the metaphysical has itself added new layers of confusion when attempting to solve the dilemma between a particle locality and quantum theoretical completeness by affirming the physical existence of a reality **assumed** (momentum) based on measurements of other presumably linked and interacting particle position. Needless to say that Einstein's strategy of maintaining locality is more appealing phenomenologically. On the other hand it would appear from the Bell theorem adoption of Bohm's measurements on spin pairing suggesting non-locality that Einstein's immanent sensory reality of experiencing locality consciously coexist with the mathematical logic of Bell's inequalities and the 'simultaneous' technological measuremens of observers miles apart! What description/explanation is incomplete? Which reality is true, Einstein's 'separability and local' appealing to phenomenological reality or the 'functionally linked and non-local' counterpart? Is it possible to modify the wave function such that mesoscopic reality becomes a hybrid incorporating both the phenomenological physical locality and the metaphysical non-locality? Stay tuned!

In a nutshell, 'self deception' during the ongoing decision-making process which had been a source of personal confusion for quite some time now, now –thanks to modern scientific technology and mathematical logic sophistications- it is no longer as threatening even though it remains as enigmatic. We have abundantly analyzed elsewhere how the human brain consciously acquires and maintains a belief 'a' tailored to the individual's present and past existential circumstances while simultaneously being consciously aware of good evidence to the contrary in belief 'b'.

Belief 'a' responds to the exigent circumstances of sheer species survival imperatives shared with other subhuman species that subconsciously also act to stay alive, experiencing neurohormonally driven psychic state of emotional feelings assisted by a corresponding good feeling of being socially accepted to share a cooperative labor with others in the community. This we had coined as the adaptive biopsychosocial (bps) equilibrium strategy for species biological survival. In an evolving reality these beliefs are expected to be modified. How much? Belief 'a', which many, including Libet, et al, thought we had no conscious control of, has been shown by fMRI to be the result of a very conscious contrivance to exist, at all costs, and why not? Do we have choices? Yes we humans do. Here we part with the beloved subhumans sharing our vital chunk of biospheric turf and develop our belief 'b'.

Belief 'b' evolves in the direct and intensity that a given subjects' intellectual resources, experiences, interests, etc. permit. It is the meditative Sancho Panza of Don Quijote's meditations that exists in all of us, constantly warning and confusing us about dangers that maybe are there or not! Belief 'a' adaptively responds to existential phenomenological contingencies along bps guidelines, a problem solver. Belief 'b' reflects on the same contingency for effective solutions today AND the 'day after tomorrow'. Beyond the perceptual phenomenological input could there be additional, non-conventional sources of information input? Quare. We believe so and have elaborated on the conceptual mathematical logic evidence sustaining our model poem. It is fair to say that sometimes we wished we had less freely willed introspective access to plan 'a' or 'b' in response to ongoing, real space time contingencies. Poor Sancho Panza having to listen to himself and Don Quixote at the same time before deciding the next step! See "Meditaciones del Quijote". I can only relate about how self-deception may represent a challenge if not an outright obstacle to self-knowledge and moral development. It is not easy to feel a stranger to yourself, consciously blind to your own moral failings while struggling to survive. Read on YOGI below and you'll get to know an embellished, fictional version of REAL experiences lived in blood and flesh.

When you meditate deep like only a 'yogi' can you discover unexpected relations, not just the mathematical logic formulation best fitting your brain storm but the unconventional beauty in form and the dramatic simplification for the prepared analyst in search of the truths they hopefully contain. The Don Quijote in Sancho Panza's brain can do more than battle fictional windmills, he can enjoy abstract beauty and reach transfinity while in search for...what? Who can ignore 17th century Isaac Newton, who dare contrive a symbolic calculus representation to frame a credible explanation about the motions of the planets around the sun! Or the deceptively Pythagorean formulation $a^2 + b^2 = c^2$ *that so brilliantly amalgamates* geometry and numbers! See [5 Seriously Mind-Boggling Math Facts]. Need I mention Einstein 'alter ego' as captured in his formulas for *special relativity*, which embodies is a whole new fancy way of looking at the cosmological multiverse we conceptualize, an entirely new vision of a dynamical evolving phenomenological 'reality?' and our relationship to it. Suddenly reality is you and your brain capacity to explain it! To make a long story short I will give you what I consider the biggest simplification about the most complex conceptualization of the sensory experience our 'alter ego' is capable of, under plan 'b'

Imagine Von Euler's alter ego genius representing the sensory sphere of our common experience as, e.g., a mathematical tetrahedron shape of four triangles, six edges (E) and four vertices (V) and faces (F). Applying pressure to its surface (F) will make it evolve into a sphere such that $V - E + F = 2$ will always be true of **any** other combination of faces, edges and vertices. Notice that any geometry, e.g., polygon, is a sphere in potency as it sequentially diminishes its size, as discussed above.This is a consistent but mind boggling fact that in such a deceptively simple formulation explains so much about our metaphysical reality. What reality is true? The ego existence or the superego dream if they both are consciously available? Are we one or the other? We submit we are both dynamically embedded into each other depending of the quality and nature of our inherited and acquired lifetime experiences.

End of Book, Part I.

YOGI

HOW TO SUBLIMATE GRIEVING PAINFUL
EMOTIONS INTO CREATIVE EXPERIENCES

CHAPTER 1

Dear Daniel, Barbie, Nini, Suzi and family you are about to read about a Rambling Chaos of Digressions to follow. Bear with me, just bragging a little, crying a lot as I continue to fight my chronic depression and grief.

Dear family. There is not an awful lot you don't already know about the circumstances of my life, but there are a few that really made a difference, which you are yet unacquainted with, those that were part of my upbringing experiences in Puerto Rico (Macondo, USA), Spain and New York. They have forever shaped my character by providing axiological insights and various relevant perspectives to choose from as my guiding torch into the uncertainties of an always uncertain future. No, it is not either about little made-up anecdotes of my ancestors, who the hell cares about who or where they originated from, Spain, African Moors, Corsica, the Arawak Colombian Indians, Barcelona or what have you. Really, who cares? Neither is it about the relative intellectual poverty and social obscurity into which I was born and bred when my mother died after giving birth nor is it about the eventual transition upon retirement from Academia to a more leisurely lake-front retirement comfort trying to share with others in cyberspace what God and my sheltered conservative upbringing had given me. For what God has especially given to you is not meant for self-indulgence but to improve the world you found according to your guiding religious faith and your faculties, those innate or acquired. And, of course, according to your luck! I don't know if my relative successes in the HiQ world is worth sharing with others or even fit to be adopted by others under similar circumstances. Maybe so. If given an opportunity to reincarnate after my death, would I reenact the same life style and strategy patterns? I am sure I wouldn't be so lucky, given the same existential circumstances I have had to cope with, including the untimely death of my uncle, first wife and my two oldest boys.

In retrospect I never expected any reward I hadn't earned by hard work and careful introspective meditation. That lesson I learned early on from Uncle Agustin Bobonis-Sierra (de la Sierra) who claimed and inherited my immature infant body soon after my mother's death, and has guided my steps throughout my entire life. He must have been crazy to add me to his other six youngens he had to feed and raise but the die was cast. He was put in my life for me to learn and follow his steps after he died while I was still in high school, a loss I will never recover from. I have been so lucky and blessed that I wouldn't have significantly changed gears or correct any major judgments on my spouse(s), children, neighbors or pets, for life is all about love and needs first and not un-affordable conveniences in that order. Stoic, sad, antisocial, shy introvert, ultrasensitive, witty, moderate, down to earth . . . , yes all of those things some loved or felt sorry about, for I never had enemies. The only thing I have missed is not being able to play the piano or conduct a symphony orchestra. Someday I hope to explain the neurological details of experiencing that quale.

Today I live dying, trying to understand, with tears cascading down my cheeks, why God chose me to experience the untimely death of my two oldest sons. I keep looking deeper and deeper into the complexities of neurodynamics for an explanation but to no avail. But here is Suzi, my good looking wife, to provide that motherly shoulder for me to incline my head on and dry my tears while our household zoo of dogs, cats, cranes, egrets, blue jays and buzzards, watch in awe both from the porch inside and the lake flora outside.

CHAPTER 2

If the reader didn't get bored with the tiresome account in the introduction, I will be surprised. Who listens to an old man talking to himself and his claimed achievements in front of a mirror, a soliloquy of sorts inspired mostly by vanity and self-serving indulgence? Such are the pleasures of a vanishing, lonely old life in the prelude of an obligatory transmigration to the unknown, the same pleasure that often resulted in productive abstractions in the past. This is a sort of creative vanity that leads you to challenge and control the impossible and the invisible. It empowers you to wrestle complexity down to symbolic or sentential logical representations you hope to communicate intelligibly to reveal their inner structural/ functional secrets. Life is an illusion and illusions are just that . . . , illusions. Perhaps I was influenced by the many worthy and inconclusive projects my upbringing family experienced and now wished me to complete.

On my uncle and mother's side, the Bobonis transplants from Corsica had played an important role in the founding of Carolina, then a palm tree haven in mid northern coastal Puerto Rico. There are many such Corsicans, now mostly headquartered in the southwestern tip of the island who could have participated in the development maybe, but they didn't. Instead they preferred to claim a special status because of their ethnic Sub-European/ Mediterranean origins, where Napoleon was born, tribal things that can only flourish in modern colonial Macondos where Indian aborigines and African slaves are still looked down upon. Many other Bobonis in the family became lawyers, professors, physicians and dentists we were all so proud of, but none like my dear uncle Agustin, who with only a high school diploma and an insatiable lust for books and knowledge no one could match, influenced my imagination. He was, is, and will always be my hero because when you combine natural intelligence and knowledge with honesty, humility, drive and high morals, nothing can destroy you. I only wish I could feel the same way about my good and handsome father's European side of the family whose push genes didn't match their own high morals and intelligence. When God gives us such wonderful gifts, we are automatically morally committed to push and improve the world we found, we have to . . . .

The most remarkable influence that dwells deep inside my mind up to this date was my uncle's claim that he was a 'free thinker', not for sale! No wonder he was simultaneously a Catholic, a Communist, a Mason, a spiritualist, wood carving artist and a tall, good-looking labor organizer, not to mention his claim as a descendant of the French "Borbones" dynasty (via the Mediterranean Corsica). He trusted me without conditions. Somehow he felt I'd follow his advices and I sure did. He lavished me with praise when I designed my first Galen radio, able to select from different radio station frequencies from a partitioned copper coil and a rotating tooth brush frequency selector design.

Leonore Mohler and Olga Iris de Leon in grammar school were my favorite girl-friends when the term meant just that, no touching allowed, and my uncle just smiled knowingly when told about my subconscious preferences during grammar school.

CHAPTER 3

Don Juan, my tall handsome father with big rabbit ears, had buried his first American (European illegal?) wife leaving their only two children stranded between New York and Philadelphia. Whether he had originally landed in New York from Spain or Bayamon, Puerto Rico was a mystery to me since I was assiduously and deliberately kept uninformed or misinformed by all about that side of the family . . . to this day! That includes my brilliant sister Virginia, the 5-year-old precocious toddler whom my good father kept all for himself while I, a premature baby, was taken to my uncle's house for care and raising, along with their other six children.

My uncle's house was not far from the infinite north Atlantic Ocean, that blue wavy vastness that witnessed so many of my dreamy preadolescent moments while lying down on the white sandy beaches, staring at the green coconuts hanging high from the tall palm trees. I scorched under the tropical sun that turned my face color to a lobster shade and my hair to look like a matted bleached rope. A Piscean by birth, I had developed a strong liking for the sea; what else was there to do after working the post school afternoons in my Uncle's wood shop? After that we had supper and was then given a thick book to spend the early evenings reading—by the kerosene lamp—about the Marxist Revolution as seen by the Red Dean of Canterbury, England, the classic "The Soviet Power".

I had also learned early to swim well, snorkel, and manage small canoes with Cecil and Cheo Nater and other neighborhood boys. I was never seen nor felt like a leader among my friends. I was lonely, sad, and dejected. Only once in a lifetime did I have a fist fight with anyone. It was a reflex response to the neighborhood's bully, Jose Manuel (Chepo) Costoso, who once noticed I was concealing a handful of coins inside my closed fist and carrying a loaf of bread under the other arm's pits when returning home from my quotidian trip back from the bakery. He asked me 'cleverly' what I was carrying inside my closed fist. As I was getting ready to innocently raise my arm, open my closed fist and show him, he whip-slapped my closed hand causing the coins to scatter on the pavement. My response reaction peaked after my frightened attempt to recover the coins, an unexpected turn of events. In retrospect, it is a recurring memory how I was driven blindly to survive my anticipated beating by repeatedly hitting him again and again in fear. He never bothered me again. Every time I left the house heading to main street, Loiza Street, to shop or catch a bus, I could feel the many watchful eyes of my sister-cousins behind me following my slow steps to the corner street before I turned. I felt loved and protected, God bless my cousins Ana, Sixta and Susana.

There is still a deep water submerged canyon area near a wharf, 'El Ultimo Trolley', where sometimes, on week-ends, I used to practice deep sea diving with a home-made pointed iron rod spear attached by its rounded end to a length of rubber from an old Firestone rubber inner-tube. My friends and I caught small marine life with the sharp spear which probably may have dissuaded Chepo, the bully, from getting too close to me? Besides, I had an athletic build, a muscular 5'6" middle stature, the result of sand papering at my Uncle's shop, weight lifting, and soccer playing exercise. That contrasted with my other personality side as a classic music collector with Benjamin Curet Cuevas, the minister's son. Once in High School I also enjoyed painting and choir singing and, all of it done quietly without ever saying too many words about it to anyone, an introvert style many still think characterizes my demeanor. This acquired attitude no doubt results from the daily lessons received about the hierarchy of values where needs come ahead of conveniences, where the content of books or people deserve more attention than the dress or book cover, where axiological considerations always come ahead of physical satisfaction, etc. Uncle Agustin was both a preacher and a practitioner. It was his pride that all seven of us children and his wife, Maria, lived comfortably, in good health and reputation, all earned through his hard labor, industry, honesty, and the grace of God.

Once in a blue moon I would meet my shy, soft-spoken Don Juan, my biological father, who dropped by for a short social visit to exchange pleasantries and random chatting. As our hearts readied to bond, we were always interrupted after a short while. There were then no hugs as I watched his departure, teary-eyed, as he slowly left our home near the ocean and disappeared in the distance . . . It was heartbreaking, and I was always left wondering why I could not hold his hand and walk with him to his house or maybe keep him with me. Why could I not leave my uncle's home holding hands with that handsome nice man my sister Virginia possessively loved so much? Those were my first confusing lessons about life and its meanings.

But, to neutralize that anguish, there was always a late afternoon when that other tall, strong, balding man that, upon returning from work, empty lunch box in hand,. he would hug me and bring stability to my quotidian life along with Ana Luisa, the oldest daughter, who cared for me and my baby needs as if I had been her own son. The circumstances whereby my father ended up in Puerto Rico from New York to marry my mother Barbara—Uncle Agustin's sister and confidante—will always remain a mystery. Everything having to do with my father was always kept a mystery. I learned recently that before he died from a gall bladder post surgical complication there was a mysterious reunion of that side of my family but I was not invited. C'est la vie . . .

Later on, I finally adjusted to that circumstance and decided to quit worrying and eventually formally ('de jure') degraded his last name to a middle initial 'O.', something that had 'de facto' already happened for a long time. I still remember many, many years back when I had held my breath in vain hoping he would show up when I graduated Valedictorian with my uncle's last name 'Bobonis' from Goyco Elementary School in Santurce. The same expectation vanished at my middle school, high school and university graduations with distinctions. C'est la vie. I only had one sister, Virginia, who my uncle always reminded me that: "She has always had A's in her school record, never a B." This warning was often followed by having me learn the Spanish 28 letters of the alphabet with colored cards soon after I was able to sustain a stable erect position from crawling! I was able to read before I walked! This made possible for me to read the newspaper before I could walk a long straight line without wobbling and falling on my diaper-covered fanny. True, it took a long time for me to walk but I could read before I walked! Cool! I remember the times when I was crawling and soiled my diaper to Ana Luisa's chagrin and scolding, just like I don't remember anytime I couldn't read thereafter.

Aurea, my pre-kinder teacher at Aponte Street, would routinely put me to sleep on a comfortable bed with a glass of orange juice so she could teach the other pre-kinders how to read. There were 6 other first cousins in my household to attend to and so it was hard on Tia Maria to care for me. But she found time to teach me the alphabet with the colored cards. Maybe that was the reason why, just before celebrating my 5th birthday, I was already in first grade. Because of my previous home schooling training, I was tested and placed in 3rd grade. I was too young and instead became an assistant and errand boy to the teaching staff who would spoil me by managing my schooling as a private student until graduation. I seldom saw a structured classroom until after graduation from elementary school. This well-meant experience would forever thereafter keep me away from structured class learning, and I had to depend almost exclusively on book reading to take my exams, I couldn't follow the classic theme presentation by the teacher and consequently I was always day dreaming in the classroom when I attended classes or just cut classes a lot. If there was no text for me to read, or if no text books were assigned, I struggled to get a B or a C in future university exams based on somebody else's class notes if and when available.

In retrospect, I believe my uncle was preparing me to retrace his steps in the advance of his socialist ideals, never suspecting I would—with my nascent free enterprising ideas— eventually influence his beliefs more than he could influence mine. When he once opted to open his own 'Sash and Door' business, I had the opportunity to soften-up a little his extreme liberal views. When I became, at the age of nine, part of his employee team, a 'voluntary' worker always fascinated with everything he said, while I sand-papered doors, moldings and windows, operated light machinery, ordered wood supplies, etc. I was in an enjoyable voluntary servitude after school and Saturdays.

At that same time, on Sundays, I was tied up with the activities of Santa Teresita Catholic Church and San Gabriel's Convent where catholic nuns trained the deaf mute children. I had the best of two world cosmogonies, the liberal and the conservative. I was becoming a moderate, a free thinker myself and somewhat of an idealist activist, of the shy variety.

During my early teen years I managed to publish and edit the Central High school newspaper, Vocero Centralino where, against the administration wishes even when we respectfully criticized curricula, budgets, etc. But the best part was when I would write and exchange poetry and notes with blue eyed, blond Nectar de la Rosa who could play the piano, dance like a sphinx and later on became a psychiatrist.

High school years are memorable, ping pong and soccer varsity player, French and advanced math classes, choir, etc. No distractions from cell phones or I-pods.

But good things don't last long. Before the end of high school, 1950, my dear uncle Agustin died, his sweet cigar fumes and his warm, bright smile gone forever. My world collapsed and as a result, I lived in a trance and felt that I, too, had died. I entered as an honor student my freshman year at the 'State' University of Puerto Rico (UPR). But shortly before then, I had tried an escape and for that whole summer I wanted to become a Jesuit priest along with Bolivar Defendini and Valentin Rivera-Guevara at a St. Meinrad, Indiana convent. When I saw those pretty convent girls and my unconscious commitment to provide my future children the fatherly attention I never got from my own, I knew priesthood was not meant for me. Today I honestly think I have lived up to that commitment. The short Seminary sojourn did not work for me and actually only Valentin eventually became a priest. I returned back to start UPR.

With the absence of my uncle provider, I was determined to become self-sufficient. So, I had also enrolled at the National Guard 482nd Field Artillery Battalion by lying about my age. The unit was headquartered in Puerta de Tierra, near the Escambron Beach Club. When activated to fight in the Korean War, I wanted to go so badly and quench my grieving pains that I began packing some things at home. However, I was not of age and was left behind after having happily packed my military gears as well. That failed plan was devastating at that time but became an important first experience in planning.

The 482nd. Field Artillery battalion and many of my buddies disappeared in action as I gravitated into my freshman university experience with the highest entrance score. Only Arcilio Alvarado and other prominent names somehow survived that stupid war. As it turned out it was meant only to be followed by the subsequent monopolistic capitalism ventures of the oil cartels . . . , my uncle's predictions still resonating today as presidential elections begin. I was lost without my uncle but my dear cousins supported me, especially Sixta who will undoubtedly become a saint and Ana Luisa.

I had scored 99% in the university entrance examination and was allowed to take choir, soccer Varsity training, ROTC and honor literature courses besides other formative courses totaling the 21 credit limits to distract me from the irreparable grieving of my uncle. I still miss him to this day more than 60 years later, but I know he is up there at Antares, that bright spot on the tail of the constellation Scorpio. When I felt lonely, I could always talk to him while I rocked my chair in the dark nights on the porch at 18 Maria Moczo Street. I have memorialized my uncle and Antares in my third published volume of "Neurophilosophy of Consciousness."

Back at the main Rio Piedras campus of the state university (UPR), I was always attracted to literature, classical music, and philosophy. Celinda, my next door neighbor and the first girl I ever especially noticed in my life, had disappeared along with my friend, Nectar de la Rosa, so I got busy. I started then to sublimate my grieving pain by trying to be productive in creative ways. I wrote an essay for a literature prize competition under Prof. Dr. Porras Cruz. Just like I had done in High School when I dared to report on a book read that only existed in my imagination because I had no time to read, when I finished my 'book report' on "El Vengador Escarlata." (The Scarlet Avenger) I even wondered if such existed in real time. This time at UPR, for my essay I had concocted a trip to a galaxy where my uncle was sure there would be found life. Camilo Flamarion's cosmological trips to other planets, the fight for a socialist republic, all inside the ecstasy of the tragic vibrations of Brahm's symphonies fascinated both of us. After a few weeks following submission and faculty evaluation of my essay, I was told I had won first prize . . . but, with conditions. They looked at me straight in my face and said I was supposed to visit the University psychiatrist 3 afternoons a week for tests and evaluations. I was deeply depressed with my uncle's loss, not unlike later on when I lost my beautiful Irish first wife, Judy, and more recently my two older sons. When will this agony come to an end? I cannot wait and harbor a death wish in my heart. Yet, there is so much left to do.

At the psychiatrist's comfortable quarters inside UPR Rio Piedras Campus, I was subjected to a battery of tests. I had failed the arrangement of the lettered cubes and Rorschard tests but had scored at the 170+ IQ level. That meant nothing to me at that time or now, it is just a potential to develop and not a label to broadcast, socialize, and brag about as it happens now at American Mensa. At that time, still a teenager, more important were the refreshment and cookies received while comfortably resting on the psychiatrist's couch, a perfect way to end a busy afternoon in college. I became so addicted to that comfort that I feigned disorientation and stress; a strategy to continue with the afternoon sessions of brownies, refreshments and accolades. It didn't take long for the 'shrink' to catch onto my trick and booted me out of the office with an approving smile of my 'loco' acting. In a departing scene, he said I would never have problems I could not handle, "you are ok," he said with a parting smile. But I knew better that there are problems you cannot ever solve, the death of your loved ones . . . .

CHAPTER 4

College time had been all about distraction from the vacuum created by my painful loss and of making enough money in the National Guard, setting up labs in chemistry, etc. to become self sufficient. After that came soccer, choir, and ROTC, no time for anything else. I had practically finished all of my graduation requirements in chemistry as a 'junior' in college and during my fourth year, I became a part time assistant lab instructor in physical chemistry with Drs. Juan D. Curet and Garcia-Morin. Meanwhile, I had applied and was accepted to medical school at Chicago's Northwestern University, and Philadelphia's Temple University Medical School, all except at UPR Medical School where I was on a waiting list. As destiny would have it, later on I became one of its professors in physiology and biophysics, the kinds of political 'things' that can only happen in colonies, like Macondo, USA.

Following college graduation, my libertarian disposition told me it was time for me to move on even though I felt my uncle's family welcomed me and would have preferred that I get a job and share the household company and expenses with them but destiny had different plans for me. I had to leave Macondo, USA and exile myself from the petty politics and social life in a colony of 'mantengo' philosophy. The beginnings of illegal immigration from Colombia, Cuba, and Dominican Republic had just started as soon as mainland USA extended welfare benefits to the colonials. This also caused a massive exodus of agricultural jibaritos to the city leaving the beautiful mountain harvests unattended. I left for New York with Cristino Colon, a real good friend, who weeks later returned to Puerto Rico to start medical school studies. He never understood how I had better grades and was still on a waiting list at the UPR state's medical school. However, as political gossip goes, one of my Bobonis uncles had taught Marxist philosophy at UPR University at Rio Piedras main campus, which in hindsight, I think was the problem. Even my sister, Virginia, questioned the admission committee's logic. Meanwhile, I worried from my temporary abode in Bronx, New York where I stayed with my brother-cousin Augusto how I could afford Northwestern University Medical School in expensive Chicago or Temple University in Pennsylvania that had accepted me. In reality, I was not sure I wanted a vocation in the medical profession where you must deal with sick people in pain showing runny, bloody, lesions and moaning as I had seen with lab animals in elementary biology which I hated. To illustrate, later on in Spain, when working at the Oncological Institute of Madrid as a research doctor on sabbatical leave from Georgetown Medical School, my beautiful first daughter, Barbara, was born. My scared wife, Judy, had already delivered 3 boys with anesthesia and the only choice available was given to me in plain Spanish, "If you want it, you can scrub and administer some pentothal yourself, just keep monitoring the vital signs." With my scared assistance to the obstetrician in charge, Dr. Botella LLusia, Barbie came into life. It then flashed into my memory what my aunt and cousins always said about my early vocations: ". . . musicians and philosophers die hungry. You have to be an engineer, a doctor or a lawyer." Life is always a compromise between conceptual dreams and perceptual realities. So be it.

After the first UPR college saga, I came back to the USA and New York for keeps, the city I had adopted, the one that saw me grow and develop as a responsible human being beginning with the co-founding of the Puerto Rican Forum to involve Hispanics in the political process. Little did they know I would end up defending workfare instead of colonial welfare and becoming a Republican with the blessing of Nelson Rockefeller. I was too proud to extend my arm begging when I could work for my sustenance instead.

I was received in Bronx, New York again by my dear cousin, Augusto. He lived there at this time with his wife and mother-in-law who didn't like me very much. They lived in tight quarters. I was too shy and broke to start making acquaintances among the young people spending time in the bars and cafes on either side of the elevated train station at Southern Boulevard, not far from White Plains. I was never a bar or a bed hopper, preferred small crowds and never talked much. Until I decided where to continue my studies, I was constantly being reminded from an Antares star above that I had to concentrate my efforts on earning money by my honesty, industry, and frugality. Without computers, e-mails, Skype, computer phones or inexpensive ways of communication at that time, I felt isolated and depressed. I had occasional contacts with my dear cousins back at Macondo, USA, but never from my father. My only friend in New York was a 60+ year old Dr. di Targiani, a philosophy professor from Fordham University, who liked chatting with me. He insisted I date Frosso Papaeugeniou, a pretty Rhodes Scholar student from Greece. I did for a while and then missed her beautiful erudite company after she had to return to Athens upon finishing her studies at Colombia University. Then I met Peter Lardis, another great Greek friend who invited me to their ocean front home at Port Jefferson, near Brookhaven Lab in Long Island. There we enjoyed diving for Long Island Sound cherry-stone clams and enjoyed Feta cheese with Huso, a powerful Greek drink. I never thought I would enjoy New York so much; Metropolitan Opera, Carnegie Hall, Guggenheim Museum, Yankee Stadium, long trips by subway at night from Southern Boulevard in the Bronx to Brooklyn and yonder, to ponder and dream. Everything was there. I loved NY and learned a lot from its people, its majesty and opportunities. I never thought my first job in New York, after being probably the first assistant chemistry lab instructor in UPR history while still a senior in college, would be pushing a cart with clothing along busy New York streets where everybody detected my Hispanic features. In colonial Macondo, USA in the 1940's, the blue collar folks were seen with class prejudice. However, watching brilliant doctoral candidates, of all accents, skin color, sex and political affiliations serving food and washing dishes at the restaurants, it didn't take me long to overcome the Spanish 'hidalgo' cultural prejudice. I began pushing my cart with pride and making lots of money in the process—only in America! My uncle was right—as long as you do the right things and behave, what others think about you is their problem, not yours to worry about!

My lodging needs in New York took me to all of the three city boroughs traveling along the famous Triboro Bridge that takes its name from its branching to Queens, Bronx and Manhattan. In none of them was I able to establish neighborly roots and lasting acquaintances. New York is in a constant state of flux and people don't get to know each other very well but always wave at you when passing by. Somehow I always had a preference for old, quaint locations where everybody knew me, my family and each other, like those in Santurce and now in Deltona, Florida.

My original Bronx location was not my choice as it was for my cousin Augusto, the hospitable and talented diamond cutter. He asked me to join his family and share their small quarters. I remembered what his father, my uncle, had done for me when I was born. Charity was heritable and so I moved in with them. At the beginning, and for a while, I was always awakened by the rattle friction noise between wheels and rails of the White Plains bound train as it applied the brakes to stop at Southern Boulevard Station, not far from 'cousin' Carmen's apartment. Many insomniac nights I would leave the building and take the dime train ride south, to the end of the subway line in Brooklyn and back, now ready to sleep. The long ride gave me a perfect solace to ponder and reflect about my next move about going to study medicine or related but non-clinical research aspects. After adjusting to the inevitable, after a while, I anticipated and really needed to hear the metallic rattle of the elevated train pass so I could fall asleep, an interesting lesson about life.

I was close to City College, St. John's University, and Albert Einstein Medical School and owned an old Studebaker (the 'old lady'). The well paid street-cart-pushing union job had ended, and I had to find a job somewhere, with live-in facilities if possible. That meant no more affordable back pack solo trips to Europe, traveling by train with no more than a medium-sized satchel. I was lucky to find work as a counselor at Irvington on the Hudson, the place of the Sleepy Hollow Ichabod Crane, and not far away from Ossining, New York where the penitentiary was located. I started my professional career as a counselor for 'Irvington House' which housed teen agers afflicted with autoimmune rheumatic fever. It was not far from the beautiful Hudson River or the rustic train station, always ready with a train going south to Grand Central Station in Manhattan. At Irvington House, I devoured book after book of anything that fell into my hands. There I met a beautiful Irish born nurse, Miss Mclooney, a devout Catholic who wanted to marry me but I was not ready. I was obsessed with carrying on my uncle's plan for me to succeed in anything by reading anything that was published anywhere.

That yearn for novelty caused me to accept a job offer as a research associate at Cornell University Medical School, Department of Surgery, located at York Avenue, the center of Yorkville, a German enclave facing the East River . . . . , a Piscean who couldn't stay away from the rivers, lakes or oceans. It was an ideal location, walking distance from Rockefeller University, Sloan-Kettering Institute (SKI), City University of New York (CUNY) and a bus ride to New York University (NYU). Drs. William Barnes and Frank Redo, my employers, were too busy with their human surgery. After learning surgical techniques used in experimental dog work they trusted me enough to carry my own research on reflux esophagitis which we published in 'Surgical Research' Journal. Meanwhile I had simultaneously completed two master-level studies at CUNY and NYU. The first CUNY thesis was done at the Biometrics Dept. of Cornell Med.

School and Sloan-Kettering Institute for Cancer Research (SKI), under Dr. Melvin Schwartz, that wonderful brainy Jewish soul. It was a mathematical thesis describing the kinetics of particle/fluid transfer across body physiological compartments using partial differential equations.

I finished the Cornell-SKI program but never claimed a diploma from NYU because I was promptly hired by SKI Biophysics Dept. located in beautiful Rye, New York, bordering the Connecticut border. I had to drive north from NYC every day along the NY thruway and was wondering how long the 'old lady' Studebaker would take it. As it turned out, it was all worth it because it was there in Rye, New York where, in a Russian class, I met Judy Sheffer, a beautiful reddish-brown-haired Irish co-worker I was destined to spend almost half a century with in company of our five children.

Working at SKI at Rye, NY was a blessing in disguise in many respects even though the highway driving and the pressure were exhausting. At that time, I was offered a full scholarship for MD/PhD studies at Albert Einstein Medical School of Yeshiva University in the Bronx. I couldn't turn down the unique opportunity to live at the Abraham Mazur student residence with those brainy Jewish people I had admired and appreciated as friends. The pressure to make decisions and the hurried married life were asphyxiating me. I had to do something soon because I didn't want to leave SKI and their superb research facilities either . . .

Probably based on my good grades and what was considered a good masters-level math thesis, Albert Einstein School of Medicine (Yeshiva University) confirmed their offer for honor registration in an MD/PhD program, room and board at the medical school Abraham Mazur lodging facility. I was elated. I had never met so many studious, serious-minded and religious people in my life. They were also very friendly with a Catholic like me. The medical curriculum was breath-taking but the class discussions were in-depth and I learned something new every day. I made good friends also, like with Dick Zackheim and others. I don't remember their names but I do remember a lady Israeli soldier turned medical student who became a close friend. Dick had a strange connection with the door entrance ticket man and ushers at the Metropolitan Opera House for Saturday afternoon operas. We could stand up and enjoy the whole opera for only a quarter. Dick and I had a standing argument as to who was better—Roberta Peters or Amelita Galli Curci. We and our Israeli friend, who was a good-looking red head (who is now probably a good physician back in Israel) spent hours together talking about the Middle East problems with Egypt, Jordan, Saudi Arabia and Palestine. Iran and Syria were not so prominent then. I often wonder about our friend's whereabouts now that Iran is sworn to pulverize the chosen people.

I cannot ever forget how, in the middle of medical school final exams, I was contacted and told that Don Juan, my father, had died. I could not attend his funeral because I had no money except my scholarship. My sister, to this day, has never forgiven me for being absent at the funeral. Confusion, guilt feelings, depression and lack of concentration followed. It was not as bad as when my uncle died, but the resulting problems with my sister's side of the family still linger. I did not take some exams and nearly failed others and was put on probation for the strictly clinical courses following. Then, my good luck made possible a special arrangement for the PhD end of the combined degree program. I would be allowed to do the research at the known facilities at SKI at Rye, N.Y. This time, instead of traveling to New York City after work at SKI, next time, after marriage, it would be to Long Island, via Throggs Neck bridge over the Long Island Sound, a long but pleasant drive along the 'Bunny Trail' path bordering the Long Island sound with Judy on board the Studebaker, the 'old lady'. The previous fun rides to New York City had bonded us and cemented our relationship and we decided to get married in cold wintry St. Paul, Minnesota in December, 1960.

After traveling by car to St. Paul, Minnesota to get married, we rented our first house in the ritzy area of Jamaica Estates, L.I., a walking distance from St. John's University main campus from where I would graduate a few years later. Judy continued working at SKI with Dr. Jacquez's cell and tissue cultures while I got very busy with Dr. Eidenoff at the SKI Biophysics lab. Judy kept working until Angell Jr. was born. She was a very supportive woman and I had maintained a good relationship with her curly, red-haired Irish mother from County Mayo, Ireland, now deceased. Her two brothers, Gene and Jim Sheffer, and I maintain our friendship to this day. In the Biophysics lab, I was given the task of designing the optimal X-ray/cortisone treatment for Sprague-Dawley rats to carry, without rejection, Rous Sarcoma tumors used variously in assays to evaluate treatment protocols of hosts carrying deadly Rous Sarcoma virus in a tumor.

Dr. Eidinoff, who was in charge of the lab., was a very busy University Physics Professor. He depended heavily on me to run the lab. Which I did by always being on time, being orderly and creative, besides maintaining a trouble-free lab. That soon changed when it became my PhD thesis research laboratory. I ran a smooth operation and made him unwilling to part with me when I decided to finish the research end of my agreement with Albert Einstein School of Medicine. When I talked to him about my new lodging facilities in Long Island and professional future plans, he offered me a deal I could not turn down. I could keep my full time job at Sloan Kettering and use all of the resources of the institution, including such niceties as electron microscopy, isotopes, and all kinds of biophysical and biochemical tools to work on a doctoral project SKI was interested in.

I was both fascinated and scared at working out the plan alone. In addition, I would be tracking the biophysical/biochemical changes in a normal chick embryo fibroblast in its transition/transformation to becoming a cancer cell, a sarcoma, after getting infected with Rous Sarcoma Virus.

I was perplexed at the prospect of following and describing how a crystalline white powder in a test tube labeled 'RSV' could become alive, infectious, and invasive of other cells after being cultured with normal cells—**Alive!!** In my original report, I had called the miraculous virus nucleoprotein a truncated life which found its complement by stealing it from the normal fibroblast host cell. Life in potency had become life in act. I couldn't wait to see that moment when life was somehow insufflated into a crystalline substance, but, as destiny would have it, the virus nucleoprotein had just disappeared while many things were happening inside the cell, as described. Not even the electron microscope could track the nucleoprotein's evolutionary grand finale. At that time the genetic code, in particular, and molecular biology, in general, was still immature and the workings of m-RNA, rybosomes role, etc. were still a subject of speculation. Who would have suspected that the viral nucleoprotein had incorporated itself into the fibroblast host DNA and there to be 'copied' by transcription and the information transferred by m-RNA to serve as a template for the synthesis of an enzyme, one gene one enzyme! I missed that but not Howard Temin whose imagination had him invoke the translation of RNA virus segment information by an unknown RNA polymerase, a reverse transcription. He used some of our SKI data to win a Nobel Prize. I was happy but disappointed and, by the time my doctoral work was finished, accepted and published, I rejected an offer to work at Seton Hall College of Medicine, Microbiology Department to further that kind of investigation.

I decided to change directions and select an area of research so complex that grants would not be so competitive to obtain and fewer people to compete with. That was the nervous system. So, after finishing the complex agreement with all concerned at SKI, Yeshiva University and St. John's University, our family headed south for Washington, DC and Maryland where research money was, even when commercial computers were not available yet. Only the federal government had such computing facility and was very much in a primitive stage, people worked inside their computers . . . . Like I would also upon arrival.

CHAPTER 5

After what seemed like a never ending trail from New York along New Jersey turnpike, my then family of three finally arrived at Sonoma Rd. in Bethesda, Maryland. Angell II, born in Long Island, NY, was barely an infant. The Smithsonian Institution was organizing a Science Information Exchange (SIE) and needed someone to handle the notices on research projects (NRP) on cellular and molecular biophysics funded by public tax monies. I was hired to handle the activities at the National Institute of Health (NIH). It was fascinating having witnessed the growth of knowledge that preceded the discovery of the DNA double helix structure. My plush office was inside a huge government computer that coordinated the scientific research activities of the whole nation. We were strategically located near Georgetown University, NIH, and the nuclear energy facilities of the Armed Forces Radiobiology Research Institute (AFRRI) at National Naval Medical Center (NNMC), George Washington and American Universities. It was fun to learn computer programming in Fortran and Basic and help develop a system to facilitate the information exchange between federal grantee researchers.

Under Dr. Foster, that amiable, tall gentleman from New Orleans, I personally handled the cellular and molecular biophysics "Notice of Research Proposals" (NRP), exchanges, and even published a magazine where virus researchers could express their brainstorms. I kept up to date with professional developments by attending conferences held weekly at NIH, across the street from NNMC and AFRRI.

After spending much time as a desk biomedical scientist writing basic computer programs and shuffling and feeding IBM cards into the computer operational system, I began missing the laboratory. However serviceable I might still have been to the Smithsonian, I felt I was just existing and going nowhere, the 'sane psychosis' of curiosity had seized upon me. Once things got organized, my professional services would become every day of less importance, as others with less academic training could run the show for less tax-payers money. So, I became a full time military officer and part-time consultant to AFRRI whose linear accelerator (Linac) was actively producing much needed material for the raging war effort in the Vietnam peninsula. I had escaped uniformed military participation before when my 482nd. Field Artillery Battalion disappeared in combat and an unusual situation came up. I reactivated my army military commission into Air Force wings that would allow me to fly freely over so many unanswered medical and scientific issues and "do my thing." The best part of it was that I could do research in civilian clothes except for summer special training at School of Aerospace Medicine (SAM) in San Antonio, Texas or elsewhere as needed. Now I was a full time researcher at AFRRI assigned the mission of isolating and characterizing an erythropoietic stimulating factor (ESF) found in hydrazine-stimulated animals whose plasma could be used as treatment (e.g., plasma expander) for injuries in the battle field. We induced anemia in sheep after provoking hemolysis of red cells with injectable hydrazine. I was happy I was not directly involved in such sacrifices which reminded me of the many dogs we had to sacrifice to evaluate the effects of a chemical I had isolated from gastric juice and now dissolved and dripped into animals with Barret's esophageal lesions or reflux esophagitis when at Cornell Medical School. I felt terrible about the animals but it was necessary I was told. Besides, the only other alternative for the dogs was death at the pound. I never suspected either that years later I would be using stereotaxic equipment to implant electrodes into living cat's brains to study their behavioral change upon selective electric stimulation. The results were verified by sacrificing animals and verifying the exact position of the brain electrodes. I am glad I don't have to do it anymore.

It was not always a rosy path at AFRRI. I had the best equipped lab in the country, ultracentrifuge and all, and published all kinds of findings on the erythropoietic activity of the fractions isolated and purified by paper and column chromatography. However, the only catch was that the results were classified and internally published, leaving my name out and crediting it to one Dr. Sigmund Baum, my boss. When I found out and politely complained, he let me know that the military felt that once the recombination synthesis of erythropoietin was possible, my GS-13 equivalent pay was excessive, and thought I should take an abatement on the non-military end of my contract.

Since I had not anticipated this development, I waited while Dr. Baum slowly grew by degrees less civil, showed boss authority which he never had before, occasionally found fault, and was ready to let me go elsewhere. Fortunately I was granted a funded faculty position at Georgetown University Medical School by NIH and allowed me to maintain a consultant position with AFRRI. In retrospect, I admit that once Dr. Marshall Nirenberg, et al had deciphered the genetic code across the street from us at NIH, it was a matter of time before genetic recombination techniques would synthesize erythropoietin in much cheaper, faster and reliable ways than the classical physical chemistry procedures I was using, as I had tried telling my boss . . . . , not that he understood what I was talking about. I tried to join the NIH team for a few hours/days to get familiar with the work going on but there were too many trying the same thing at that time. I saw it coming, and when I realized it long before it happened, I knew I had to change gears. My biophysical chemistry research, interesting as it could have been, was destined to become obsolete and I would be expendable. I thought I would try teaching 'molecular physiology' to medical and graduate students at Georgetown Medical School not so far away.

I accepted a grant from NIH to do some membrane biophysics research which I combined with my teaching. I told Dr. Baum that I would not compete with him for a position at the Armed Forces Medical School in Bethesda, Maryland, that his wish that I find an opportunity to work on the nervous system was unnecessary, for I would leave that instant and stop at Georgetown University Medical School where I already had a job waiting for me. Dr. Larry Lilienfield, Head of the Department of Physiology and Biophysics was waiting for me.

To my chagrin, I later found out that Dr. Baum's offer to give me a good recommendation anywhere I went was tested only to find out he praised me but warned that I may become too independent, a free thinker, something deemed not so good in team research. My opportunity to land an NIH group job in Puerto Rico disappeared on the warning about me being an indomitable 'free thinker', like my uncle had been. I had forgotten I was referring to life inside super political Macondo, USA.

CHAPTER 6

When at Georgetown U. Medical School, I was finally doing what early on I had thought was my vocation, combining research with teaching. And I was really happy being married to Judy, that beautiful Irish red head. None of the girls were born yet but three boys kept her plenty busy in our brick house with an acre-fenced yard in Kensington, Maryland. It was not far from Rock Creek Palisades, as we discovered later on, when water began seeping ever so slowly into our huge basement office.

The pay from my NIH grant and basic faculty salary was not bad and allowed me to gradually pay off the debts I owed for my successful allergy desensitization and constant billings from the pediatricians. Things were looking up but, like my uncle would say, "Always secure your credit and character as a serious-minded person, be truthful and always make your word and last name your best assets." I took care not only to be in reality industrious and frugal, but to avoid all appearances to the contrary, and I made sure I never caused scandal and paid duly for what I bought. I can say today that I can die in peace knowing that all of my children were transmitted and assimilated the same principles of Christianity and fair play. It helped that nowhere in sight were places of idle diversion. It is true that we never went out golfing, fishing or shooting because our three boys were too small and Romeo, our huge Great Dane filled our hearts. A fellow professor from Georgetown sold us a cat to keep Romeo company, but the cat turned out to be crazy and we had to return it. Romeo was relieved. Angell Jr. was overactive inside and outside his crib and sometimes pounded on his brothers, Johnny and Daniel. Who could have known that many years later that six foot six inch, 200+ pound Navy electronics expert son would be confined to a wheel chair depending heavily on both of them?

At Georgetown Medical School, things were developing slowly. My course in 'Molecular Physiology and Biophysics' was too biophysically oriented to attract many graduate students and even less medical students as electives. I joined one, Dr. Allen, in developing a bioelectric cell. He used chemical solutions, but I was more familiar with the cellular mono-layers growing on a glass surface like the ones I had used when at SKI. The glass was now replaced with a platinum electrode surface and connected to a voltage recording apparatus to measure the current output and power generated as the cells grew inside an experimental, special media. Later on, I would present my results at the Biophysical Society Congress in Moscow and Mexico where I was received royally.

In the middle of the cold war, when I arrived in Moscow, I was assigned an academic escort/interpreter. I did not know Russian enough to carry a conversation, ditto for my escort in English nor Spanish so we settled for "Pig German" and plenty of body language. Wonderfully, I was able to attend the opera house to watch an unbelievable ballet performance of Tschaikowsky's "Swan Lake." I also attended mass, where Eastern ritual was not unlike the Catholic equivalent I was used to in the west. To my surprise, I was invited to fly to Akademgorodoff, (City of the Academy), Siberia where all eastern important research was done. There I did three unforgettable things: Placed my signature on a special library book, collected stones along the shores of the largest existing Lake Baikal, and made a long distance call to my wife, Judy, on the other side of the world. Angell Jr. received a shoe box full of the beautiful stones as a present.

I realized that I did not feel satisfaction doing such bioelectricity research because while I was becoming more sophisticated with the various academic disciplines I had to be familiar with, I saw no marketable practical application in sight. I knew that soon the NIH funding would be revised and I would have to again shift gears.

I received an opportunity to get a sabbatical license and was invited to work at the Oncologic Institute in Madrid, Spain. I combined my experience at SKI and Georgetown and would try growing rapidly-dividing cancer cells on Platinum electrodes. By doing so, I could either increase the output of the bioelectric cell and/or learn more about the mysteries of the cancer cells, the same ones that years later took the life of my dear Judy to heaven. So, on to Madrid with wife and three boys . . .

The airplane trip to Madrid from Dulles Airport in Washington, DC took more than 13 hours traveling with the three boys and a TV set which I kept under the airplane seat. It was a nightmare trying to control toddler Angell Jr. Everybody was happy when the airplane landed at Barajas Airport outside Madrid. We were supposed to stay for a few days lodging at a motel until contact was made with the Oncological Institute. After an overnight stay with Angell Jr. antics, we were told it would be in everybody's best interests if we left the motel. With the help of an employee of University of Madrid Medical School, we secured a nice fifth floor apartment on the road to Asturias, near Madrid. We spent many nights trying to keep Angell Jr. from the windows and wondering if we should have sold the house in Kensington and left our Great Dane behind. Was that a sign that we wouldn't return to Georgetown until NIH grant renewed or disappeared altogether? Or was it possible to stay and work in Madrid? But working where, doing what?

Francisco Franco was still in power in Spain, and we witnessed his gray uniformed guards ('los grises') beat up medical students to the ground without their knowing what the provocation was, as alleged.

The research plans for an academic visitor on sabbatical leave were not clear. Helping technicians and personnel took siestas following their narcoleptic big lunches until 2:00 P.M. and then worked until 10:00 P.M. when their supper was light. Research was slow in Spain, but the basic science background of the medical students was far superior to their counterpart in the U.S. The opposite was true for the clinical training which was not as organized and effective as in continental U.S. ('Conus') America. Only the well 'connected' got the opportunity to make rounds and see patients with the clinical stars of the different departments. We had three occasions to test this. First was when Angell Jr. developed a fulminant fever that required his tonsils to be removed stat! I couldn't believe we had to wait in line with other kids to have tonsils removed by an ENT specialist armed with an intraoral device to cut the tonsils out without any anesthesia other than ice cubes given them to taste while they waited in line. He nearly bled to death! Having that tonsil vessel branch cut so close to the carotid artery was a big risk to take. Poor kid!

The next experience was almost as risky. I mentioned this before, but it is a memory I won't ever forget. My wife, Judy, was ready to deliver Barbara, our oldest daughter. She never had any serious complications when delivering the three boys, except Angell Jr. in New York. After a period of sedation with a mask connected to sodium pentothal, delivery was safe. At that time in Spain, women pushed, grunted, and yelled when delivering a baby. Judy was ready to take a plane back to the U.S.! Dr. Botella Llusia, the leading obstetrician at the time said, "Well, we have epidurals and we can provide the sedation but you have to set it up yourself. You ARE a doctor, aren't you?" I was petrified and sweated blood. I had a lab coat on, put some sterilized gloves on and a nurse helped me mix the IV drip and set it up to provide the sedation. Soon after that, there came that gorgeous madrileña I had also helped to deliver. Barbie was born!

Last but by no means least, a crazy idea came into my mind. Since my research was not advancing very much, blaming the institutional siestas and all, maybe I could get the sabbatical leave to count as the equivalent of an internship and take the medical license exam. I had all the course work. Then I could practice medicine instead. The brainstorm did not last long. One Dr. Baena, an Asturian Internal Medicine professor from the University of Madrid Medical School agreed to let me follow him in his rounds, ask questions and participate in the discussions. I hated to deal with bleeding or infectious patients. I was reminded of my first undergraduate biology course when my professor insisted on my taking a live frog home in a shoe box so I could play with it during the weekend to get rid of my fear and pass the class. My theory exam grades were very good. The real test came one day when after examining a cardiac patient with a stethoscope, we noticed the characteristic dry sound heard when liquid accumulates between two surfaces, the endocardium pressing hard on the contracting heart and the pericardium. The pericardial effusion had to be identified first before the fluid could be removed with a needle through the pericardium into the cavity avoiding perforating the endocardium into the heart cavity full of pressurized blood that would rush out on contact with the needle. "Don't be afraid," Dr. Baena's high-pitched voice would repeat in a fatherly way, "You will notice that the plunger in the syringe will start coming up as it fills with clear pericardial fluid. Just wait. Then when the syringe fills up, it's easy." I thought to myself, scared to death, "Like hell it is." I took my lab coat off, never again to make rounds with Dr. Baena or anyone else, I swear.

Everything became very frustrating, except watching Barbie grow in Madrid, before returning from the sabbatical back to my NIH grant at Georgetown Medical School in Washington, D.C.

While in Madrid, I never had the chance to meet and visit with Jimmy Ortiz, a West Point graduate and dear friend from high school who—at that time—was stationed at the U.S. Embassy in Madrid. But I had occasional contact with his friend in Puerto Rico, gynecologist Dr. Benjamin Curet, a buddy I had spent many hours listening to classical music with when growing up and who had connections with everybody. Being the son of a minister and member of a distinguished family of university professors, it was easy for him to recommend me for a faculty position at the medical school there. I had worked as an undergraduate assistant and lab instructor to his brother, Dr. Juan Daniel Curet, a Professor of Physical Chemistry at UPR before. Besides, the prospect of transferring my NIH grant to UPR made me more attractive as a candidate. If Georgetown U. opposed my leaving the position or demanded a reimbursement of sabbatical expenses, then I had to look again for a house near Georgetown, near the DC area. This uncertainty about a professional future would have been solved had I followed the prevalent materialistic approach and practiced a profession and got rich but, somehow, I felt my call was to investigate and assist in the formation of intelligent minds to lead future generations. Not that I detest the perks that come along with wealth, it was never my first priority. But I had to be practical and do whatever was necessary to sustain my beautiful family. My first academic priorities could perhaps wait until I retired when I would write for myself and share with anyone interested . . . . which I have done . . . . with no riches attached but with many controversial brainstorms, as the case may turn out to be, circulating around the HiQ communities for discussion and analysis.

CHAPTER 7

Once I became a regular faculty member at the state University of Puerto Rico Medical School, it made me feel odd. Here I find myself now as a professor at the same institution that put me on a waiting list when other more prestigious universities had accepted me without hesitation, but c'est la vie. Never look back, show your class, and labor hard. My uncle was smiling from Antares out there in the Scorpio constellation. Because of my biophysical background I was expected by Dr. Pinedo, head of Physiology and Biophysics Department and my boss, to join Dr. del Castillo at the Neurobiology Institute in Old San Juan where ionic fluxes across artificial membranes were being studied under voltage clamp conditions, among other things. My mathematics master's thesis on the kinetics of flow across body compartments would become handy. As God would have it, my NIH grant at Georgetown University was not transferable to another institution and there was not enough money around to set up a lab for me. So, full-time research was out of the question. I had to spend time there with Dr. Pinedo's intestinal absorption studies and with Dr. del Castillo's membranes, when not lecturing or running the physiology labs.

After work, I drove back from the then medical school building, next to the San Juan Capitol building, to the Valle Arriba Heights cul-de-sac in Carolina where my beautiful 5 bed-room house for four of us was facing a big park and made me relax, especially when the calm, relaxed demeanor of my wife took the stress out of me.

Since our youngest daughter, Denise, was not born yet, everybody had their own private room. I felt proud that I was living in the town my Bobonis side of the family had founded years ago. My cousin, Papo, who owned an iron works shop, had transformed my spiral art design into protective iron doors covering the entire front of the house.

Meanwhile the state university system was expanding and new campuses were opening across the island. The then president of the entire university system, Don Jaime Benitez, had somehow learned about my research frustrations, and my administrative abilities and unfulfilled dreams when I had set up the research lab at AFRRI's Department of Defense (DOD) facility and asked me if I would be interested in becoming a co-founder of a new university campus in Cayey, way up in the mountains of Cordillera Central where the old Henry Barracks military installation during the second world war was located. Judy was expecting our fifth child, Denise, and that would be an ideal place to raise a family. A colleague of mine at the medical school had singled me out as an ideal candidate to evaluate his new vasectomy procedure. It worked out, because Denise was my last child. To Cayey we went, along that sinuous mountain highway of so many memories, the 'Autopista'.

Then, there, in the middle of that inter-mountainous valley, I was offered a strong brick house where the command officers used to live, all paid up, housing and utilities, as 'combat pay' for leaving the city and coming into that natural paradise where all of my five children grew up to become, in my fatherly-biased mind, the best citizens any nation can produce.

Thereafter, life was always a challenge. I had all the possible administrative positions academia could offer, from advisor to the university president, to Chairman-Dean of Natural Sciences faculty, to Biology Department Head. However, I felt unable to effectively influence, in my typical non-political ways, the need to abandon that submissive colonial life style and choose liberty, either as a banana-like republic sans resources or a State of the American Union. No government would ever grant Puerto Rico the idealistic, tax free, Commonwealth status without having all states of the union claiming the same pipe dream status. Life in colonial, political Macondo, USA can be asphyxiating, the reason why, upon retirement, I went back into voluntary exile in Florida, USA. I had to. This was to be the unique chance in a lifetime that would give an idealist like me the time to influence the formation of future generations of great men and women while marketing some of my crazy ideas on the brain dynamics of self consciousness.

At the same time, shaping and helping to improve the character features of young minds attracted me. This way, I would create consciousness of the importance of both public and private domains and how to avoid the excesses of both communism and monopolistic capitalism and their common greed for power and money at the expense of the involuntary needy. This also was a unique opportunity to provide the guidelines for searching for the pathways leading to the source(s) of righteousness by self-education. The monopolistic capitalism preached upon false principles. Greed had to be displayed as a clumsy exploitation apparatus pointed at a false goal, leaving the citizenry destitute of the proper just means/criteria of comparative axiological principles and becoming prepared for a reasonable course in life where priorities are properly assigned by man's private powers through education. No doubt it should be invaluable in influencing the correct early formation of the individual character because it is in youth that we plant and later harvest our good and bad habits and prejudices and decide what trade or profession, pursuits, and matrimony suits our personal circumstances. What starts well ends well and if we are consistent, it will become the education of a wise man incapable of being turned into the cruel politician or professional warriors so damaging to the human race. The rules of prudence in ordinary affairs are learned first at home and developed while young. It is with the interaction with your fellow students that you learn not to be ashamed of your Taino, African, Arawak or European origin and you will be forever convinced of how unimportant all/any origin is to happiness, virtue, or greatness. As Dean of the Faculty of Natural Sciences, I required that the most experienced professors include a course in basic sciences and spend time in shaping those young minds to be prepared for their eventual appearance upon a world stage. The means to achieve the proper goals then and later are as complex or simple as wisdom allows. Thus, we can choose either content and enjoyment as opposed to being stressed and tormented by regrets or regrettable impatience. We need to regulate our minds by practicing frugality, temperance and diligence.

During my busy schedule investigating, lecturing and administrating, I found time to lecture on Neuropharmacology and Neurophysiology at the Ponce Medical School in southern Puerto Rico. I also wrote a monthly editorial column for the local newspapers in Spanish "El Mundo," and English "San Juan Star." I hope my own children understand why I had so little time to exchange tete-a-tete daily dialogues with them except on weekends when all seven of us occupied a whole pew on Sundays when attending Catholic mass in Montellano area of Cayey. It would be proper to say that the Cayey experience provided the multidisciplinary background so useful when attempting, upon retirement, to model a biopsychosocial frame into which existential reality could be better understood. Besides publishing two textbook volumes on Human Biology, I had managed also to publish at Editorial Limusa, Mexico, the basic elements on a biopsychosocial (BPS) model of consciousness that later on, upon retirement, would expand into 4 volumes on the "Neurophilosophy of Consciousness." I spent every free minute inside my office at the mountain university, looking at Cuco, the bull statue that decorated the entrance to the old Natural Sciences building, and reading library books which afforded me the means of improvement by constant study. I also set at least a couple of hours each day for peaceful, isolated meditation. The geographical isolation of that beautiful valley in the mountains, Cayey provided the kind of setting conducive to a reclusive life that kept me away from taverns, games, and frolics of any kind. My commitment to have the best undergraduate Natural Sciences faculty in the whole UPR system continued indefatigable, besides my higher commitment to a young family of five gorgeous, healthy children growing up to be educated in the future.

Judy was a very studious person herself and would never complain about things most people would, a stoic attitude that worried me. But, it was indeed lucky for me that I could count on her as another one much disposed to intellectual growth and frugality as I. A cell biologist herself, who later successfully completed a law degree in Spanish, not her native tongue, was commendable. We studied together and became lawyers at the same time. She assisted me cheerfully in the discussion and evaluation of many a brainstorm regarding my limited research activities with students or curriculum design. Her constant reading of philosophy, her minor *concentration at St. Claire College in Minnesota, was seen by our children as a bold and arduous project of arriving at moral and ethical perfection. I, personally, had to depend on my natural inclination, upbringing, custom or enterprise activity and how it might influence or lead me into rightful decisions.

As a faculty dean, the undertaking was at times more difficult than I had imagined. Dealing with prima-donna professors coming from the United States, North, Central and South America—and many from Spain-, made me realize I had to be very careful because of cultural sensibilities. To be completely virtuous was not sufficient to prevent our occasional misunderstandings. This meant biting your tongue, avoiding controversial military habits that had to be broken and substituted for good interactive civilian ones also acquired and established. With my wife's constant help, I was able to gradually depend on a steady, uniform rectitude of professional academic conduct. That never stopped me from always behaving like that shy, reclusive and idealistic loner many a times taken to be a snooty, conceited knight riding on his high horse. But I never abused my high positions. It was tempting at times to remind the science specialists, especially mathematic experts, that they also had to be cultured into other humanistic areas so important in the transformation of young students into well-informed and effective future leaders. I designed an 'integrated science' curriculum where all professors were invited to participate and were required to root their contributions of science content in their historical evolution to the present time. Many colleagues hated the idea of having to update their knowledge on how things were, how they were presently, and how they were likely to become. In the process, knowing they were dealing with college freshmen, they had to hone their essential virtues and, not only master the content, but face the challenge of a clear transmission to un-experienced young minds. This required a good dosage of fortitude, industry, sincerity, moderation, justice temperance, order, chastity and humility. In my personal case, after five children, I had to concentrate on industry and frugality precedence because of outstanding debts, and the need for saving for rainy days. I had been thoroughly trained at and exposed to the rest of the virtues at my uncle's house. Needless to say, with the advantage of hindsight, I never arrived at the perfection I had been so ambitious in obtaining for others, and in fact, a few trivial bad habits hardened and became incorrigible. But the fact that I tried, by living an exemplary life with all of my family, influenced others, and it was later recognized with university plaques after my retirement.

All of my children grew healthy and happy inside that Cayey faculty 'country club' as many envious local residents chided. Security gates, 24/7 guard protection, swimming pool, free house and utilities and a beautiful landscape, and of course Judy, was a gift from God.

Angell Jr., the tall, oldest child, was finishing high school across the street. His entrance exam for the state university was "number one" for the region. His same high record was obtained for the Asvab Navy aptitude test. Little did I know that, upon graduation, he had it all figured out to accept special electronics training by the Naval school in Chicago. I drove him to the airport soaking my shirt with tears. We were a close knit family.

When time came for the rest of our children to go to college, we moved back to Carolina, but this time to a three-story, fully-equipped and furnished building with an outside office, where we lived, worked and also rented. There was a beautiful office on the first floor from where my wife and I practiced law. I would handle the medical malpractice cases part time because I travelled daily on the highway to reach the university campus in Cayey while our kids went to college. Johnny was attending Hotel Administration School, Daniel went to Architecture School, Barbie specialized in Plastic Arts at UPR, and Denise earned first prize Valedictorian in high school and then registered as an honor student at UPR, following in my steps. Meanwhile, I was exhausted travelling many miles back and forth along highway 52 to Cayey, lecturing at Ponce Medical School, writing articles for two newspapers, writing a book, and preparing and litigating cases.

Like her older brother Angell Jr., Denise developed 'wanderlust' and went to the University of North Carolina in Greenville, North Carolina as an exchange student. She earned her Bachelors Degree in Kinesiology there as a regular student. That left Daniel, Johnny, and Barbie in our household to care for while they finished their university degrees at the University of Puerto Rico.

What Judy and I considered an extended family Hispanic-Irish tradition, was later on, upon returning back to the continental U.S., considered as an over-protective strategy that would interfere with the ingrained North American tradition of self sufficiency 'out of the nest'. Meanwhile Angell Jr. continued travelling all over *the world aboard a US Aircraft carrier, and Denise completed her studies and eventually had a short-lived marriage to a local, wealthy North Carolinian. As the political situation in colonial Macondo, USA turned intolerable, and still is, we couldn't wait to return back to the continental U.S. We built a lake-front home in Deltona, Florida where I still live.

I was not ready for retirement and couldn't find an equivalent university position in Florida, so my family went ahead of me, and I became a commuting professor between Deltona, Florida and Cayey, Puerto Rico. I couldn't wait to return to my family and stay there. I missed them terribly. I counted the days until retirement every day but maintained an expensive transatlantic telephone conversation with wife as often as possible. The only one to be affected by the move to Deltona was Johnny, who was only able to finish half of the 4-year Bachelors Degree curriculum in Hotel Administration sponsored by Cornell University at UPR. He would have preferred the Hispanic way of life. This was in sharp contrast to the time when, having moved to Puerto Rico from the U.S., he did not understand a word in Spanish. While taking classes at a catholic academy under Ms. Santa-Pinter, an Argentinian teacher, who wrongly thought he had some learning problems, he was forced to sit in front of the classroom on a high chair for everyone to laugh at. This was a cruel experience that affected him to the very end of his shortened life.

Before designing our beautiful lake-front house in Deltona, Florida, Daniel was doing architectural design work for Zalloumco Construction, a custom-made design challenge where he developed his fine architectural skills. He and Angell Jr. were the first ones to move into our house after Angell had accumulated overdoses of Ibuprofen which ruined his renal function. At that time, the cold war was raging, and after leaving the navy, he was gainfully employed by a Washington, D.C. based Martin and Marietta Company in support of the cold war effort. When the cold war froze, he lost his job and his incapacitating health problems began.

The unprecedented Middle Eastern problems and global awakening were brewing, and the quality of life began to decline. It turned out to be so for almost everyone else in sunny Florida, where all white elephants traditionally come to die.

CHAPTER 8

I had no idea what was waiting for all of us in sunny Florida upon retirement. I was lost without a secretary, a lab assistant and without any experience or ability for cooking, mowing the lawn or keeping a house account. Judy had spoiled all of us and now she was not feeling well.

This frustration was picked up in my first medico-legal novel in the English language, "The Duplex House." There I describe the early stages of a transition from a busy productive professional life to a busy but non-productive home life. After being interviewed and offered a job as a Social Security judge in Orlando, Florida, I was ignored when they found out I was a card carrying registered Republican voter. I then found a job lecturing Anatomy and Physiology at a University of Central Florida (UCF) campus, and now Daytona State College, to keep up with the rapidly evolving field that applied to the brain. Also, the rapidly developing computer technology satiated my appetite for knowledge anew.

There were many family health problems to solve, but I was not intimidated by the seeming magnitude of the undertaking ahead of me. Fortitude and forbearance always work great changes and accomplish great results if one first develops contingency plans. Amid all these evolving health problems, I had plans of going back to my first vocations as an undergraduate—philosophy and music. I would again become an industrious and frugal recluse and, by cutting off all dolce-vita amusements and other employments that would distract and divert my attention away from the execution of that dream, I had promised myself to develop as a life plan a theory of self consciousness. My original plan to continue the piano training I had started early on with famed pianist Carmelina Figueroa at the free music schools (Escuelas Libres de Musica) failed. It failed because, while the theory was relatively easy, performing now and then felt like I was using 10 cramped thumbs. So I continued the collection of symphonic masterpieces I had started at age nine when one song would fit into one side of the hard plastic disk and later on a symphony fit into both sides of a long-playing record. Now we have many choices at Internet music radio.

As Angell Jr. continued living with renal-failure complications, it was very hard for me to watch my oldest son suffer, and I donated one of my kidneys to him, a drama described in "The Duplex House" novel. Judy had recovered from her breast cancer removal and chemotherapy and was enjoying life in our beautiful 7 bedroom house by Lake Louise where I still live.

I pondered about what better thing I could do than follow the path my destiny had traced for my mission. This mission my uncle had expected me to follow, whatever that was, in which he trusted I would excel and make my contribution to posterity . . . . if possible. But first, I had to get acquainted with Deltona and some of its then few hundred inhabitants.

India Boulevard was empty and our house was built after they put a post light in front of the only other existing house along the boulevard, across the street. Deltona was an unincorporated piece of land, a bedroom community for Orlando, where everything happened in Central Florida. So, before I dug in I began now to turn my thoughts to community affairs, beginning with health, utilities, public safety, and available jobs for my adult children. I joined the community council that preceded the now controversial City Council initiated a couple of years later when Deltona became an incorporated territory under the leadership of John Masiarschik.

Deltona today is the largest city in Volusia County with almost 90 thousand inhabitants, no major industry, and full of spoiled youngens and politicians-for-sale. On the whole, we were satisfied with being established here in the boondocks even though we regretted there being at that time no provision for a hospital, college for a complete education of youth, no civic organizations nor supermarkets. There was a church on practically every other major street and a good library. The Deltona Inn, near the exit from I-4 corridor, was the only place of entertainment. West of Deltona, across the I-4 corridor, was Orange City and beautiful Debary which followed the contours of the St. John's River on its sinuous and meandering path to the north into the Atlantic Ocean at Jacksonville. Before its trip north St. John's River separated Volusia County from Seminole County's Sanford Marina to the south and Lake County on the west side. To get to know the community I renewed my membership with American Mensa, rejoined the Knights of Columbus near our parish, Lady of the Lakes, the Rotary Club and the Elks. These same organizations had provided in Puerto Rico a safe social outlet for our family to socialize and we hoped for the same outcome here in Deltona.

We were active at the Community Council and it didn't take long for Florida Fish Memorial Hospital to set foot nearby at Orange City and the Daytona Beach Community College (now Daytona State College) to flourish as the city didn't stop growing. Daniel was establishing a good name designing expensive houses for the growing areas surrounding Deltona. Angell Jr. was in a stable condition working as distributor for a major company and Johnny worked as an apprentice assistant manager with a pizza company while Barbie designed flower displays for a Loews store.

I then embarked on a follow-up on my previous publication with Limusa Editorial, Biopsicosociologia. However, I was lost trying to adapt to life in Central Florida, a long shot from what our family had experienced in NYC, Spain, Bethesda, MD or Puerto Rico.

There was something different in the sociology of Deltona that merits mentioning and explains our surprise at seeing so many churches when we first came here. All kinds of different church denominations, including the catholic church in different locations, were busily involved in community building, from assemblies in the open air subject to bad weather forecasts to meetings inside closed old buildings where persons were appointed to receive contributions destined to procure the ground and erect the definitive building, where the congregation was to meet in prayer and important community work. Isolated communities always have unemployed labor, broken shop-keepers and several other insolvent debtors, including several illegal immigrants of indolent and idle habits, or paroled out of crowded jails. If you were not in the health or fast food industry, there was little to do except clearing land, cutting cane, or peddling illegal drugs. Deltona was pretty clean in that respect. Preachers of the Baptist faith were pretty good in running their charities and always made large collections. Their down-to-earth, grass roots eloquence had a wonderful mesmerizing power over the hearts and purses of the congregation, wherever assembled.

Judy, after a double mastectomy from cancer just before my retirement, began showing signs of a relapse that would finally take her away and precipitate my tragic emotional downfall as described in my second medico-legal novel written in English, "The 15th Sunday of Extraordinary Time." From then on, I felt just like I did when my Uncle Agustin died. The floor had fallen from under my feet and I was freely falling or floating in space. After almost half a century with the same good woman, one can never forget. As Judy's health progressively declined, all my children began drinking more often, and this may have contributed to Johnny's ongoing hepatic ailment that confined him to an involuntary sedentary life of disability and eventual untimely death.

When I got really involved with my wife's recurrence of cancer and my growing investigation of brain dynamics, I had to disengage myself from city and county affairs, especially after I had tried to run for the City Council of my district and withdrew once I knew someone else was also running for same District 5. Besides, I felt I had earned and secured some leisure time during the rest of my life for philosophical studies and family amusements. I purchased a fully equipped computer with all peripherals and software perks, and proceeded in my "thoughts experiments" with great alacrity. But, as is natural, my family and close friends now often laid hold of me for their medico-legal problems, at times imposing some duty upon me to investigate or draft a document which I dutifully complied with.

CHAPTER 9

At the time my dear wife, Judy, was not improving after her breast cancer had returned with a vengeance, I was also getting ready for donating a kidney to my older son. My youngest daughter was having marital problems and my oldest daughter left our house in Deltona to join her in Greenville, North Carolina. I had to get my mind busy to avoid being mentally crushed by my own emotional feelings, like I feel now after the untimely death of my two oldest sons. Deep concentration isolates you temporarily from your existential problems. Besides, I had been for some time now preparing myself to synthesize my ideas on reality and consciousness upon retirement. I thought I could pick up inherited genetic DNA memory, perceptual sensory input, acquired memetic memory, conceptual inferential input (based on language processing), and the associated emotional mindstate all into one comprehensive hybrid biopsychosocial (BPS) physical/metaphysical package embracing the physical ontological and the metaphysical epistemological, and weaving it together by the quasi deterministic glue of quantum theory that left room for free will and a credible explanation for self consciousness. A big project indeed! I would avoid mentioning my Catholic religion because I was convinced it was not necessary, and I could use the same arguments non-believers use to prove my point and be more convincing thereby. I was determined to prove that a belief in God was subject to rational logic analysis as a strategy for biopsychosocial (BPS) survival as a species. Somehow we had to escape the classical dogma that only the human mind sensations and rationality constituted the exclusive cognitive faculty. I had to find what was in between, how the sense-phenomenal **"perceptual"** input was coded into general neuronal network representations expressing the universality of the otherwise direct, singular objects/events immediately presented to our senses in the environmental niche and how their corresponding **"conceptual"** inferences also find their way into general neuronal network representations expressing the indirect, mediate, attributions and explanations about their meaning to the body economy in the biological, psychic and social (BPS) spectrum. The search for meaning was to be found with the aid of language sentential or symbolic logic representations making possible the co-generation of self-consciousness and the associated mental state corresponding to the particular judgment in relation to the sense-phenomenal (internal or external) input, genetic/memetic memory input, and their associated emotional mental state. Ideally, each input would be dynamically and globally integrated and the resulting package would be dynamically updated and be retrieved from cortical attractor spaces on short notice as our adaptive judgment on a given contingency. Sensibility to the body proper "internal" and the environmental "external," as a bottoms-up process would now include not only sense-phenomenal intero, extero and propioreceptors inputs, but also transfinite inputs into quantum electromagnetic energy absorbers like DNA or RNA! I was spreading myself too thin until I would asymptotically get to know everything about nothing. The heads-down process of understanding the meaning entailed the emergence of self-consciousness with the help of the silent inner proto language generated in the language processing.

I was convinced that what has escaped the imagination of most of my colleagues has been the realization that both the perceptual input, bottoms-up and the conceptual, heads-down processes are severely limited in their content and capacity for resolution in our human species. Thus, when making judgments about optimal adaptive spatiotemporal responses to important contingencies, we can no longer have certainty about the truth value of our input or output content or meaning respectively, we only have probabilities. We have no choice but to satisfy that human innate curiosity about our origins and destiny and make mental representations of that micro subplanckian and macro cosmological invisibilities with the aid of metaphysical epistemological logic tools and cross our fingers. Ergo, the ontology value of an un-aided scientific methodology is complemented / supplemented by epistemology because understanding and sensibility are both subserved by the faculty of modeling with a hybrid epistemontological approach which I had promised myself to develop. Thus, incomplete in the absolute sense as they are, the practical reason that Kant defended must be now reinterpreted to include evolving explanations on the structure/function of the invisible, non-existential reality that includes theological and physicalist faiths. The cognitive processing undertaken by the rational faculty depends on the quality of the bottoms-up information to produce the logical inferences underlying our head-down modal judgments, hopefully consistent and coherent, within the context of our biopsychosocial existential reality. And this is necessarily reflected in our evolving legal codes and constitutions. It is clear that the self-conscious affirmation of one's existence, the "I" actor and observer, is situated at the executive vortex where all relevant perceptual/conceptual representations converge as the synthesis of the several semantic constituents of that cognition into the high order cognitive singularity content in a cortical premotor attractor space ready to be consciously chosen to activate the corresponding muscles or glands into executive adaptive action. How these primitive representations in the form of a-priori logical constructs are assembled within the existential circumstance and ongoing mental state of the subject and made available for free will access and choice may be outside the reach of rational tools, and I anticipate much trouble examining what I consider the most crucial human cognitive faculty. The most difficulty will no doubt be to explain the induction of the self conscious state with the language faculty and assigning a cooperative role to synaptic and electromagnetic quantum processing.

It's a brave new world we are all witnessing. The comfort of the quotidian existence under the Boolean world of truth or falsity and certainty has evolved into the stressful uncertainty of a statistical probabilistic world where disjunctive and conditional statements always enter the decision-making process to preserve the truth-functional structure of logical reasoning. Many of us, whose hobby is to model reality, have to always keep in focus that our most serious brainstorm pronouncements are necessarily inferences on representations and never descriptions of observable falsifiable reality. In the bottoms-up phase, our brains represent inner and outer objects and events inputs for linguistic processing into other types of metaphysical logic representations and the heads-down output are only inferences, only representing a mediate cognition of that original object/event. Our particular judgment on a given situation, i.e., our opinion, is thereby the result of representations of previous representations until one final concept binds many representations and worse, many concepts may comprehend a single representation. Our judgments are far from being objective. They are inferential and subjective. That is the best our species can offer in the matter of cognitive certainty. That fact of life when combined with another fact of life, our innate curiosity about our species origin and destination, necessarily makes room for beliefs and faiths, theological, physicalist or whatever. I had much difficulty marketing this unpopular idea among non-theists. Not less difficult was my attempt at developing a convincing formulation where I had to settle for the simultaneous cogeneration link between proto language (inner language) processing and self consciousness as just a convenient explanation for the invisible processes outside my limits of corroboration as to the details.

Marketing these concepts to multidisciplinary audiences is most difficult, especially when dealing with theoretical physicists and mathematicians who would not accept that their physicalist constructs are in themselves 'beliefs' not radically different from classical symbolic or sentential logic representations leading to belief-type 'propositions'. These latter types can be as fallible and uncertain as the former and, considering their intended influence on social conviviality, both may be considered as subjectively necessary and sufficiently unfeasible propositions. Ultimately, they are both the result of unconscious genetic, subconscious memetic processing of bottoms-up inputs (from internal and external objects or events) into neuronal network representations, including their assignment of agreed-upon language-related label descriptions or attributions predicated on their size, shape, color, etc. to be followed by conceptual elaborations predicated on those or related previous representations of same objects/events in memory. At this level, the functional copula subject-predicate (object/event description or action, e.g., table is red, chair is moving) allows for the formation of logical language rules according to which judgments are expressed in a logical syntax and semantic form necessary for communication in a given language. Ergo, both propositions and beliefs are ultimately inferences about an invisible world derived from the use and application of pure laws of logic and expressed in a predication copular format (subject-predicate, modal-conditional). Coetaneous with the modifications leading to the final structuring according to truth-functional value considerations, a self conscious identification with such circumstantial consideration ensues. In this respect, I took issue with Chomsky's syntax-semantic vector in formulating sentential logic. They defended the vector based on the primacy of the innate primitive biological self-preservation imperative 'meanings' ('intension') controlling syntax considerations. They neglect the influence which depend on the idiosyncrasies of the adopted language structure. Curiously, the actors behind the recent advances in technology have given low priority to issues only capable of being expressed in modal or conditional logic formats, especially when the brain's emotional states, resisting logical formulations, exert a causal influence on the outcome of a decision to act or not. Somehow physical theoreticians seem to conveniently ignore the inexorable presence of real life existentialist component (emotions) in every significant human judgment. Unfortunately, it is not so much about the legitimacy of a rational, truth-valued, unified composite of objective, meaningful and relevant parts defining a claim about the ideal world as much as it is about how the lonely leader and his emotional mental state circumstance will translate into the needs of the society he represents vis-a-vis his own. The logically structured, semantically well arranged, truth-valued judgment representing the best legal and moral, biological, psychic and social interests of a collective is only a goal in clear controversy with the biopsychosocial needs of the individualized components of the collective. All propositional 'facts' or theological 'beliefs' are of necessity inferences about the visible and invisible aspects of existential reality, life inside an epistemontological hybrid reality we cannot escape from. Ergo, existential reality does not exclusively equate with objective reality. The former is an acceptable, subjective constraint of reality in se whose absolute truth and meaningful values are only apparent. On the other hand, how accurate and 'objective' can the human brain representations of objects/events be? Especially when further constrained by the imposed linguistic compositionality in which it must be expressed in both inner and reported modes using the subject's proto-rational syntax/semantic straight jacket. Thus, claimed 'objective judgments' thus elaborated are not to be confused with the symbolic or sentential logic **"truth"** of their representations as materialist physicalists would have us believe. Logical consistency is a necessary but insufficient part of the totality. Symbolic or sentential logic representations of the invisibility of the noumenal or cosmological reality can be rationally intelligible yet truly valueless. "Truth" is a goal to be achieved as we travel the sinuous path along an evanescent asymptotic line. Consequently we can only have opinions on the **probable value of our representations** of an invisible reality, and that is as close as we can go about knowing the truth of our absolute reality. We can only aim at an isomorphic correspondence between the structure / function of an object/event and the symbolic/sentential logic representation as expressed in a syntax/semantic copula we call an 'intensional' explanation or opinion, not a description which we reserve for sense-phenomenal entities. This means that the brain cannot produce absolute truths whether analytical (in differentiating), synthetic (in integrating) representations before the facts (a-priori) or after the empirical facts (a-posteriori). For all men and rabbits all empirically based, synthetic judgments (a posteriori) are the result of subconscious processings and can, in theory, be programmed in a computer. They relate more to the guarantee of biological survival of the species as they interact with a potentially hostile phenomenological environment with limited necessary resources. At the exclusively human level where psychosocial considerations become part of the survival equation we have to resort to, brain representations of the chaos of sensations, and access an innate language faculty to classify, sort, combine, permute and parse to extract the meaning of an otherwise atemporal, acausal and asymmetric reality 'in se'. Genetic and memetic memories of past and present provide the bottoms-up input of coded representations to evolve probable alternatives of adaptive responses to future contingencies to be freely chosen by consent from pre-existent dynamic probabilities in a cortical attractor space reservoir. In the process both language and self-consciousness are cogenerated. The participation of the amygdala, hippocampus, thalamus and limbic system in the formulation and synthesis of the representations (in harmony with natural law) into neocortical phase spaces has to be detailed and remains as a great challenge to cage into a credible formulation. The materialist physicalist need not be challenged by a hybrid, epistemontological model of reality because, as Kant admonished, conceptual thoughts without perceptual meaningful content (intensions) are empty just like a pure physical ontology without a metaphysical epistemology is blind. The indelible complementary/supplementary and semantic interactivity of perceptual and conceptual (ontology, epistemology) is of the essence for an existential cognitive act to take place, for neither senses can conceptualize nor rationality sense.

However, all human species limitations in perceptual / conceptual resolution being considered, it is fair to say that there may be conceptual meanings without rational underpinnings (intuitions) or perceptual experiences that resist their formal expression as logical constructs (revelations?). Should they be considered empty, bogus or meaningless and denied cognitive status? Just like quantum theory—nowadays the best 'scientific methodology'—cannot qualify as being exclusively and **objectively** valid, it is nonetheless rationally intelligible about the invisibility of a subplanckian reality containing massless 'objects'! Unlike this case, theological theist experiences cannot be combined with ontological measurements to generate quasi objective valid arguments as is the case also with brain dynamic modeling. But recorded history and human experience of negentropy has validated the anthropo-centered, self-referential non-conceptual intuitions we know as religious beliefs. The Cartesian type of truth preferred by materialists would leave no room for scientific or religious beliefs in that it requires the actual sense-phenomenal verification of the object/event being precisely reduced to symbolic/ sentential representations in its physical absence. Beliefs, by and large, are defeasible and subject to evolutionary modifications. Moderation requires that beliefs be subjectively and objectively sufficient and coherent with sets of other beliefs. In theory propositions may be false yet the believer—theoretical physicist or mystic—can demonstrate that his conviction is operationally justified until revoked in the lab or in the social ecosystem niche. The embodied finitude of the human species condition justifies more cognitive flexibility. And this includes a consideration of the inseparability of the human emotional affect at all stages during the elaboration of a final judgment, a very difficult element to include/formulate into the equation. The judging capacities of the existential human being in his circumstantial milieu cannot be ignored by self-serving purists. I hope this emphasis on human existential realities is not construed as a free willing Sartrian type of existentialism. It simply means that the logical format of Fodorian 'propositional attitudes' formulations has to emphasize more on sense-phenomenal content at the expense of self serving logical format. But, for the purpose of communication we need to categorize ongoing sense-phenomenal perceptions within the framework of an agreed-upon universal a priori referential for the purpose of providing guiding rules for the evaluation of objective truth content, freed—when possible—from irrelevant modal or affective 'non sequiturs', reminiscent of the Kantian 'Categorical Imperatives' controlling the participation of fallacies and moral sins in the formulation of propositions. It may be necessary to psychologize modality in the structure of the subject-predicate copula if it helps identifying the semantic content of a judgment. It is difficult to distinguish propositional attitudes from logic modality. A predicate monadic logic concentrating on 'intensional' content is sufficient for our limited purposes of a brain quantum dynamics model.

It is important to realize that, because human existential reality is in the brain, an understanding of its dynamics must start with the raw data of sense-phenomenal impressions, in the style of empiricist philosophy. But these sensory impressions are limited in conveying information about the structure/function of existential reality. So to compensate for ontological deficiencies in resolution we need to complement/supplement the paucity of facts with an epistemological rationalist approach based on credible meta sensorial, probable but defeasible / revokable facts as found in metaphysical logic propositional representations, as stated above. After all, not all cognitions arise from sensory data but also from innate genetic memory, acquired memetic memories or a combination thereof. The epistemological component of the 'hybrid' approach I am suggesting will accommodate whatever logical procedure there is available that brings you the closest to an original sense-phenomenal description. This may take the cognitive format of substituting the invisible 'form' for its visible 'effects'. This transition from a sensory 'description' (what) to an inferred 'explanation' (how) as an acceptable identification has two modes in their order of reliability: logical and natural supervenience between the invisible object/event X and the credible manifestation of its inferred presence by logical induction or a measurable and falsifiable effect Y. How does an invisible X relates/determines Y? Ideally one can isolate X logically but not in nature. X will have a strict causal determination of Y iff X features are necessary and sufficient to generate Y features such that changes (form or semantic content) in Y will cause a corresponding change in X. In brain dynamic studies we have only a limited number of ways of establishing the relationship between the X variable of interest (e.g., anger, interest, inhibition/activation, etc.) and Y a measured (increased circulation, metabolism, electrical activity, etc.) or behavioral effect (crying, laughing, etc.) as a function of a controlled input (sensory/ environmental or spoken/semantic) by the investigator. When these a-posteriori cognitive responses are elicited in the absence of sensory impressions we suspect they respond to innate or an unidentified a-priori input. So long as mathematics is a valuable language tool to represent objects/events in their absence or 'represent' other representations, semantic judgments, a-priori or not, depend on their original tangible content and not on the language tool. It should also be noticed that sensory modalities are neutral and only the circumstantial reality of the actor makes them meaningful or not, as registered in the output/behavior.

CHAPTER 10

It took some time for me to finally realize that retirement was an entirely different ball of wax when making household decisions. I had to adopt an entirely different mindset to see and effectively interact with wife, children, pets and their old and current controversies 24/7. Now there were no secretaries, assistants, student helpers, etc. to help me run my ship and enjoy the pleasures of a leisurely plan-ahead for the content of new courses, labs, curricula and other perks. This was a new world I was not prepared to adapt to, least to lead. This feeling was reflected in my afore-mentioned medico-legal novel venture in the English language, "The Duplex House." To make things worse, at that time, my wife was getting worse from the cancer chemotherapy onslaught and my older son was ready for a kidney transplant. How can any retired human being suffer like this and still be able to sink into the deepest levels of conceptual abstraction? This was reflected in my Volume I of "Neurophilosophy of Consciousness" book where I essentially outlined the various possible routes towards understanding the problem I was about to tackle and never really resolved. You can practice wingless flying over the fence or your neighbor's house, but you will never take off from your lawn except in the virtual reality of your dreams. Soon after I donated a kidney to my son and lived through a near death experience after an intoxication with an overdose of an opiate, life became a via crucis watching my saintly wife slowly dying. Even the heavens protested when four hurricanes visited us in Florida soon after she finally died at the lake-front house where she wanted to be for this moment of transfiguration, our hands firmly held together until hers lost their grip and I held my breath. Judy had passed away . . .

That Christmas, I spent seven sleepless days and nights fasting with peanuts and red Pinot Noir and writing, non-stop, my mea culpa novel "The 15th Sunday of Extraordinary Time." I dedicated it to that great Irish lady who gave her life to raise my five children and bring out the best of my feelings and creative potential. Soon thereafter, all my pets died also, and I wished I could have joined her in that special abode she must have in the highest of virtual heavens. We all still miss her and know she is looking down, watching over our three remaining children and her idealistic Quixotic husband that was. The more depressed I felt, the more I needed to get involved in abstract theoretical insights that would mesmerize and capture all my attention. I also underwent psychological treatment during my bereavement at the local Hospice facilities.

CHAPTER 11

After being married to my first wife for forty four years, I was devastated when she died in July 2004. I joined a Hospice Support Group that met on Saturday mornings. There were nine of us who met and shared our grief for an hour each week.

One hot summer Saturday in August, 2006, we met a new member of our group, Suzi Beauchamp, who had lost both her son and husband in January of same year. She walked in wearing a white sun dress that I will never forget. Even though she was also grieving, she had a great sense of humor and complained about the terrible coffee in a joking way that brought laughter to our group. After hearing her tell of the two deaths she had recently endured, I decided immediately that I was drawn to her and wanted to take her under my wing to help her. The following Thursday, I called her and asked if she would like to go with me for a sandwich at the Florida, Deland Elks. She hesitated and stated she wasn't ready to begin dating but I said, "I'm not asking you for a date—just a sandwich. You have to eat you know." She finally agreed and that began our complex but happy lives together. We were married the following October 2007 at my house with our support group and intimate friends and family in attendance.

When Suzi became my second wife, an entirely different but necessary chapter in my secluded but safe cage opened in my life. I would come out of my sheltered cocoon and face real, unsheltered life. Meanwhile I had already finished and published the Volume II of the series "Neurophilosophy of Consciousness, An Epistemontological View of Reality." Could I abandon my search or continue my obsession with trying to make a path as I walked? Would my new wife accept my isolation and my bigamous life with my computer-wife? I tried to answer some questions on quantum-based brain dynamics, and in the process, there came more questions to answer than I had bargained for when I started. Would Suzi, that outgoing, beautiful fashion model from North Carolina and Virginia, ever understand the silently grieving, shy, conservative loner? A carefully groomed and fed veritable household zoo of dogs, cats, birds, ducks, egrets and other lake-front mammals, and every flower, bush and tree growing inside and outside the large house would keep her distracted from me and her own family issues . . . . most of the time. Meanwhile, I continued my grope brain dynamics studies in between emergency health problems with my two ailing sons, Johnny and Angell, Jr., who were then living in Daniel's house on Sullivan Street in Deltona, Florida. Daniel had been deployed to Iraq, another constant worry for all of us even though this time he was a specialty consultant for the Department of defense with no other weapon than a folded newspaper when walking inside a terrorist infiltrated compound! Difficult times indeed.

Suzi was the complete opposite of my first wife, Judy. She was an extrovert, always finding something to talk about, outgoing with our friends, and absolutely unable to sit still and relax. Judy was quiet, a homebody who was afraid of having company in our home. She loved to read and was content to be with her family. Suzi brought friends over for dinners, loved to go dancing, sang karaoke, and loved people. She brought two cats with her but added two more plus a dog. At first I was. exhausted trying to keep up with her, but I finally realized that she had opened up a new world vision to me that I had not known before, and 1 began to enjoy and learn new things in our new life together.

Since Judy had been sick for several years before her death, our house was in much need of some TLC. This was Suzi's first priority. She began painting the rooms and redecorating everything in sight. She had brought her own furnishings from her house when she moved into my house and began blending hers with mine, a feat I had no clue would work. But it did. Then she started on the yard and landscape, sometimes working into the darkness to finish a project. She and her son, Don, wall-papered the bathroom and she bought new mirrors and fixtures for that. I was amazed at how nice everything looked. I teased her about making our home into a "museum." Suzi had several collections—bisque doves, Pillsbury dough boys, tea pots, dinner bells and many figurines and "dust collectors." However, she managed to incorporate them into her decorating scheme that appeared uncluttered and tasteful. As l worked on my computer, I watched her in action and was exhausted just observing her energy and expertise, now somewhat diminishing as aging and morbidities encroached upon her.

At one time in her life, Suzi had been a fashion model and had also owned her own florist shop. She had also had some rough times during her early years that she often talked about. She had raised three sons and prior to moving to Florida, had attended nursing school and worked in the hospital in Fredericksburg, Virginia, and also had worked in a couple of doctors' offices. In addition, she had done home health care and been a caregiver to her mother and ailing husband all at the same time. She also worked in a florist twice a week just to "play in the flowers" and enjoy the respite from all the family sicknesses.

When she moved to Florida, she began teaching school part time as a respite while she was caregiver to her husband who was dying of prostate cancer. Her husband died January 11, 2006 in Florida, two weeks after she buried one of her sons in Virginia.

In December 2007, Suzi's mother, now in her 90's, was suffering from very poor health in North Carolina. We brought her to live with us against her mother's wishes and Suzi made her last months of life bearable and fun until her death in April, 2008. I was then able to see another side of Suzi, her caring and loving soft side that had not been so obvious to me before. This same Suzi became my rock when my two sons became so ill prior to their untimely deaths in 2012. She mothered all of them. She continues to "mother" all of our pets, from the indoor pets to her "outdoor" ducks, cranes and birds. When one of her mother ducks was killed by a car, Suzi helped another mother duck raise 37 ducklings in 2009. Pet food controlled our marital budget as it became as expensive as our own food. IRS would not accept pets as dependants . . .

At this writing, we are both still grieving our losses and occasionally escape out to dance and enjoy our friends. Suzi has slowed down a little and has discovered that being retired means doing some of the things she always wanted to do but never had time for. We have traveled a little, something we both enjoy, and settled into a life of more leisure. I realize that I have been greatly blessed by the two wives in my life, each one opposite from the other in character but similar in the things that really count in Christian living. It was time to continue with my neurophilosophy investigations.

I had previously been warned about the technological explosion of the post computer, late 20th century age, and the cognitive strangle-hold theoretical particle physicists had on controlling science/natural philosophy evolution into the 21st century. I always liked to stand on solid firm ground before my mind soars into the virtual domain of open-ended abstractions. In real life, a good car mechanic may be more important than the physics professor. specialized in auto mechanics when it comes to fixing my damaged real car. In the study of consciousness we have many problems to solve in the physiology of the brain even before we understand how it works as a causal mind executive. But theorizing about how the mind processes sensory input and executes an adaptive solution transcends the immediate and sets the strategy for solving ALL putative and related problems that may arise. But you still require hands-on knowledge about the structure/function of the car/brain the way a mechanic/professional does. When, upon retirement you work alone and when this search is translated into mind/body relationships neither the bright logic mathematician nor the skilled neurosurgeon alone will perform in a satisfactory way unless you go multidisciplinary and constantly fear spreading yourself too thin. But it was better than knowing everything about the computer formulations applicable to brain dynamics by studying more and more about less and less until asymptotically you knew everything about nothing! Anyway, it was going to be hard multidisciplinary work but I needed the challenge to escape my emotional pain and chose the super complex hybrid epistemontological way. This decision required choosing the logical foundations of my 'existential' approach. My conclusions would hopefully be falsifiable in the laboratory measurements and/or verifiable on the metaphysical logic desk. Ideally my judgments on self consciousness would be of the synthetic a-posteriori variety leaving to mathematicians the analytic a—priori computer processing of their symbolic/sentential logic representations which did not require their familiarity with structural/functional aspects of e.g., the amygdala, hippocampus or cortical columns. Likewise, knowing about them and not knowing what to do with them other than excising them or injecting some specific medication when injured was not the solution either. We had to develop a hybrid approach combining their respective contributions into one whole unit, the epistemontological unit.

We needed a synthetic a-posteriori modus operandi to be based principally on empirical or contingent results of varying degrees of generality. Our species sense-phenomenal resolution limits underdetermines sensory impressions as to their truth value and semantic content. Consequently, the resulting judgments are based on empirical, not a-priori, intuitions. The logical truths of analytic judgments includes those possible worlds in which human experience in those noumenal worlds is impossible. Their semantic contents is conceptually, not sensory based.

It is important that we learn more about brain dynamics, about how we humans make decisions on important and relevant biopsychosocial (BPS) issues that control the quality of our quotidian and intellectual lives because human rationality is essentially oriented towards making continuous adjustments to optimize the outcomes of our interactivity with changing environmental influences beyond our control. Because of the self evident biological imperative for the human species survival, as witnessed by the spontaneous, unconscious servo controlled adjustments, our efforts are biased towards an anthropocentric focus sustained primarily by meaningful and trustworthy empirical/referential data inputs. Thus the emphasis on formulating our judgments based on synthetic a-posteriori propositions especially when analyzing the relevant psychosocial aspects of existence where the results may not necessarily be applicable in all possible worlds. This is not meant to stop the search for universal synthetic a-priori truths as a goal when budgetary priorities are assigned. If nothing else, we unavoidably come to the conclusion that beyond sensory phenomena there 'exists' a complex structured reality that resists being reduced to logical representations. All languages explain this as being caused by an 'intelligent design' without being committed to a spatiotemporal description. While natural philosophies are systematically built up on propositions whose bottoms-up inputs originate from directly referential sensory attributions perceptual data, or their conceptualized representations, our innate self conscious faculties generate a higher order unity that requires the consideration of an 'intelligent design' as history and self-evident negentropic order testifies to. Is there a non-rational or proto-rational consciousness that transcends empirical existential reality? Quare. It was always fun to search and maybe identify the equivalent explanations within the context of biblical Baptist conception of reality which my wife Suzi, an ordained Deaconess, strained to explain as bringing stability and order to most common folks. She had her feet on solid existential reality! She made clear to Quixotic me that windmills cannot substitute for real existential problems.

CHAPTER 12

Many retired colleagues and friends from academia often wonder why would anyone like me insist on continuing to spend precious retired family time trying to explain things like life, consciousness, language acquisition and processing, brain neuronal representations of information and their translation into both inner and reportable language, etc. Is it not better to spend your unpaid time during retirement in sports and entertainment at the golf course or at a bar? Why this almost obsessive, compulsive search for explanations about an invisible world at both ends of an infinity spectrum? Does the mind hallucinate when burdened with a hypothesized overabundant supply of gray matter? I mean also hallucinations on messianic ambitions or on controlling minds for universal or self-serving benefit? I never paid much attention to this slow but unrelenting drive to analyze, scrutinize and forever search for a reason or explanation for anything and everything that moves or not. Or was this all an escape from continuous mental pain sublimized? This is enough to drive anyone normal out of their minds to experience or witness on a daily basis. If not, ask my pretty wife, Suzi, always moving around solving her family's unemployment or health problems in perpetual motion along the fast track style of her existence. All of which makes me think about what proportion of doers and thinkers society needs for survival? Can our Volusia County drivers survive without Suzi-like auto mechanics . . . . ? No! Can they survive without Yogi-like experts in classical auto mechanics theory . . . ? Definitely yes! Should people be free to choose their hobbies after retirement? Some choose to be entertained, bar hopping, playing golf, stamp collecting, bed hopping, writing, lawn landscaping, reading, cooking, playing music or travelling. Some choose to be informed as a hobby. What could be wrong with marrying your computer in a joint search for invisible objects to be arbitrarily represented with letters, numbers or words so you can now play with them using also arbitrary and convenient logical rules of play? Should that be considered a hobby or a psychopathological behavior sometimes termed 'sane psychosis'. Should we be saved from enjoyable psychic, indulgent self destruction . . . . ? Suzi reads, does civic work, writes well when inspired and tends to her flowers, curtains, ducks, egrets, dogs, cats, . . . and me. I have joined many civic organizations for a long time, Rotaries, Elks, Knights of Columbus, VFW and attend two churches but must confess that my almost exclusive interest was not civic but rather to provide a secure environment for my growing family to socialize. Except that I am considered an antisocial loner where shyness is often confused with conceit until I get past either 2 glasses of Pinot Noir or 2 shots of Haig and Haig Pinch whereupon I join the social group, relax and share my corny German jokes with the yawning, un-interested rest. If I dared to exceed that liquor quota of liver poison, I returned it back to mother earth in convulsive, uncontrollable bouts of oral greenish recursive jet ejections. Then Suzi would drive our Nissan new Altima back home while my head hung outside the car window to inhale fresh air and resuscitate. But before I go to bed I religiously check my computer for exchanges, comments or replies from the Mega International, Omega, Prometheus, Mind and Brain, WedConscious, Ispenet, and other 'one in a million' HiQ listings I participate or monitor, all worldwide groups specializing in all aspects of brain dynamics. All before closing my eyes while giving thanks to my virtual God of choice for all blessings conferred upon me, family and neighbors, nation and earth . . . Not surprisingly, I have to re-read the listings again the next day. Then I find that, e.g., Leon, a brilliant computer engineer, who had been urging me to consider his theological ABC model brain storms as relevant to my interests in developing further my BPS model of consciousness, was dead. I had the urge to reply:

"Dear Leon Maurer (now dead), wherever 'you' happen to be now, ... if anywhere., I have been considering your invitation to unite your offer to join your ABC and my BPS models and abandon the quantum theoretical probability interpretation I now follow. I admit that other than modifying a little the Cramer and Walter Freeman's transactional models to accommodate my neocortical pre-motor attractor phase space fixation, I have not been able to cover the details by using micro quantum theory at the Planck level of organization even when my modification is partially rooted on Freeman's brain noise background amplification of sensory signals and subsequent resonant phase coupling with ongoing brain activity. I believe there is enough in quantum theory to justify exploiting its possibilities to adequately represent a reliable picture of thought/language generation that accompany the attainment of the self-conscious state. We may have to invent a new physics to deal with the relatively more reliable measurement of atoms and molecules in fMRI, etc. For example EEG values may represent a spectrum of preferred frequencies varying as does the value of cells membrane's resting voltage and/or ionization potential."

What I was trying to tell Leon, the genial mystic, was that we need to spend more time with solving real-time problems here on earth, at the mesoscopic level before we spend all our energies and focus in intergalactic other world's mystical issues. We need not to abandon either the cosmological nor the subPlanckian invisibilities focus, what we need is to bring those conjectures and speculations to bear more directly into human health, psychic happiness and social conviviality, i.e., pay more attention to the real needs of real people in their pursuit of an individualized, fitting biopsychosocial equilibrium. What this and other considerations suggest to me is that to make sense of it we may need a radical new approach where condensed dark matter, Compton length scales and quantization of Planck constant may have to be considered to bring quantum theory to the macro/mesoscopic level of analysis where it may properly belong. This will allow for a better understanding of how the genetic memory encoded into DNA/RNA influences the activation of unconscious reflex adaptive responses as mediated by the amygdaloidal complex. The 20 A-acids synthesized in response to novel sense phenomenal input may represent the first steps in the production and/ or activation of the relevant membrane receptors in hippocampus where context analysis of the original stimulus takes place. The dark ionic supra currents and their quantum character may be responsible for the phase transitions observed but it would have to be established that the value of Planck constant can be quantized to harmonize it with the observed frequency value range in EEGs. By the way, if you feel I may be dreaming of dark matter instead of a white Christmas, or have exceeded my Christmas quota of Pinot Noir or Courvoisier cognac, I will understand! ☺

But one has to pay close attention to dissident expressions because it could indeed be the case that ALL of human knowledge is relational. As, what is cold without heat, light without dark or good without evil? Or as they say, perhaps conscious free will and unconscious determinism, structural/functional order and random chaos, sense phenomenal and ESP virtual reality, are simply different propositions about the same arguments of scientific logic?

As we confidently sense the solidity of an inert gold ring with our fingers science tells us that, not only that a solid ring consists mainly of empty space, but also that inert objects, such as gold rings and rocks, consist of particles whirling round each other trillions of times a second!

Likewise, as I have repeated so many times, we are ALL believers in some entity we may want to call God, or not and all may be right, just "traveling the same circle in opposite directions." Because what is God if not a symbolic conceptualization of perfect order and harmony? History has recorded myriad conceptions of God since the dawn of civilization, from the monotheistic God of Judaism and the Trinitarian God of Christians to the non-theistic Buddhism. In fact, the characterization of the same conceptual God of order and perfection comes in all JudeoChrIslamic flavors and yet vary so widely that there's no clear consensus on the definition of the exclusive God that different theologies claim, including materialistic 'atheism' belief in a strictly corporeal (material) world with no afterlife remnant. The classical believers believe God has an incorporeal (immaterial) existence, and that there's an afterlife.

As I have repeated many times, my BPS 'epistemontological hybrid model' of existential reality incorporates both material and 'immaterial' aspects as being essentially a co-relative unit. This is another way of saying that "Life and consciousness represents one side of the equation, matter and energy the other." This is not to deny that the current scientific paradigm is properly based on the belief that the world has an objective observer-independent existence, including the human species. But observers we are, only that our sense phenomenal experience as observers of ongoing objects and events depends on our brain, no brain, no reality. We build our understanding of its perceptual and conceptual aspects based on the known limitations of our human species to resolve the details of their noumenal mysteries, a pitiful state of affairs. Consider for example the foundational base of our most successful scientific tools, quantum theory, e.g., the double slit experiment.

When you watch radiation particles pass through two slits in a barrier, they go through either one of the slits. But if you don't watch, they go through both slits at the same time. And one may properly ask how can a particle change its behavior depending on whether you are watching it or not? So we invent the waveform as 'representing' the particle to explain the simultaneous passage through the two slits. Just an explanation like Suzi explains what she couldn't witness but it makes some sense when we witness the consequent results of their invisible presence. I still think there is a difference between particles mass—however small—and their attributions, the latter being its mode of propagation as a wave. Who knows?

Life is much more than the interactive collisions of some atoms and molecules. Space and time are just convenient tools of the mind to measure observable changes in shape, form, location, etc. of objects/events inside our 4-d existential cage. Likewise, how can their separated quantum-entangled particles appear instantaneously connected on opposite sides of the cosmos as if there's nothing separating them? And how can events in the present effect those in the past? It has even been claimed by scientists that particles sent into an apparatus(?) could retroactively change events that had already happened in the past. One wonders how other species conceive space and time, the properties of matter, life, etc. Does reality mean different things to different observers? Ultimately, is life just autogenous motion and change perceptually intuited but only conceptually comprehensible? But motion is a change in position. The human mind invents the concept of 'time' to measure change and 'space' to measure the displacement from an original position observed. This way, the mind can best understand e.g., the concept of 'velocity' (cm/sec) as uniform displacement in position (cm) every unit of time (seconds). Ditto for non-uniform displacement as in e.g., acceleration seen as a change of velocity (cm/sec) every second. Thus the mind uses relational conceptualization of perceptual events and comes to the intuition of the 'excluded middle', i.e., a perceptual object cannot **be** and **not be** at the same time and space. Due to our species perceptual limitations we **feel** the living presence of relevant entities in our lives that escape sensory detection and thus we intuitively **conceive** the possibility of an exception to the logic of 'the excluded middle' and thus conceive of the presence of a living, but invisible, God that has provided the foundations for theologies to build on according to their spatio-temporal circumstances. But to some believers God is more than a relational concept product of a complex brain dynamics. For theological believers there is an afterlife. For atheist believers death is the irreversible change/end of any conceivable 'life' as we know it (motion and change of perceptual matter). This self-imposed myopia leaves no room for the possible existence of relevant objects/events that exist below the threshold of perceptual sense detection, e.g., the living survival of invisible condensed matter (below Schwartzchild radius). There is no reason in the world why one should choose to ignore any and all possibilities just because there's has been an evolutionary break in the continuity of space and time upon death. Is it more logical to conceive of a single particle passing through two holes at the same time? Or like 'biocentrists' claim: ". . . you can consider yourself both alive and dead, outside of time". Is this to be considered a logical violation of the law of the excluded middle? Or do we just simply die and rot into the ground while the cosmos continues to tick along like a clock until it reverses its expansion, growing hotter until everything is crushed out of existence in the conceptual possible 'crunch'. This Big Bang→Big Crunch→Big Bang oscillating cycle of 20 billion years duration is part of the Buddhist worldview.

The classical view on the conservation of energy in a hypothetical closed system where the resulting increase in the order and complexity of the finished product. i.e., increase in free energy (F) is at the expense of the decrease in the other energy component (-E) of the totality (T) according to T= F + E. Entropy energy (E), besides being equated with an increase in structural/functional disorder it is also considered by some as a transformation into its equivalent matter (M) state according to $(M = E/C^2)$ not available now to do work inside the close system but available as an ingredient to a contiguous synthetic component system (a consumer predator somewhat analogous to a link in a food chain where life will continue in the starved predator at the expense of the 'dead' prey). This interpretation would be valid if the special consumer-predator is identified. What it means is that we witness the causal chain of linear progression resulting in what seems like a spontaneous increase in organization and complexity (a decrease in the entropy of the system or negentropy) and nowhere to be seen the predicted energy fuel source to drive the counterintuitive increase in complexity. To say that there is a source of energy in an open system is an act of faith just like describing the resulting complexity as being caused by an 'intelligent designer', whatever that may be to any observer. This is a logical, and not a theological, argument as many of my detractors argue. In the absence of such physical identification, a metaphysical explanation may do and call the designer =X. In ancient Greece X were Gods of lightning, thunder, etc. Today we jump into the truth train and ride along the asymptotic railway to Noumenoland to measure the natural events or simulate them in the lab. As we get closer the dubious/nebulous certainty of our sensory descriptions soon become the probable and then the possible truth as we struggle with the sentential or symbolic representations that our limited combinatorial brain processor can handle. The asymptotic train trip from the ontological certainty wish station → epistemological probable/statistical stop → theological possible/intuitional stop → "I give up" final stop describes the genetically-driven human angst in identifying his origins and destination. The serious limitations in our sensory and computational brain hardware pretty much predicts that life will remain an asymptotic journey to Noumenoland, never reaching that destination.

A similar frustration attends our frequent analysis of the 'life' fact. It was not spontaneously produced, as defined in thermodynamic theory for the organization of complex systems. It required a source of external free energy to fuel and sustain physico-chemical reactions resulting in the resultant living organism. It resulted in an increase in structure and complexity of original organic reactants leading to the living organism result. Life cannot be described as a random, blind process according to thermodynamic theory. It was caused, driven by heretofore invariant and unidentified forces responsible for the particularities of the end result. It describes a causal chain of linear progression resulting in a decrease in the entropy of the system (negentropy) environment where such event took place. The eventual structure/functions (of proto-life) are influenced by both genetic and physical/environmental conditions (nature) present where such events took place. The eventual/future structure and function of living descendants (in sexual reproduction) is predicated on parents reaching reproductive maturity and procreating; what we call evolution by natural selection. We can argue that evolution by natural selection (henceforth Mendelian determinism) operates at both the level of the ontogenesis of the individual immediate parents and a recapitulation of the phylogenesis of their descendant(s); what we call evolution by natural selection. Thus, if energy is constant (cannot be created/destroyed) and entropy may be considered a form of energy not available/free to do work, then the total (T) energy may be described as a sum of free energy (F) and entropy (E); T= F+E.

Consider that when, e.g., heating an egg white there is an expenditure of external energy as the egg proteins denature and become tangled, that is also explained in classical physics as the transformation of the viscous, amorphous liquid egg white into a structured solid with a determined dimension and shape requiring heat energy to attain that particularized end configuration. This is an endergonic process, arguably just like creating a particularly beautiful solid statue from an amorphous viscous cement pile requiring the energy and imagination of the creative artist. It is argued both processes would still require additional 'energy' to further change their configuration, e.g., a push from the window to reduce the statue to rubble or a grinder to reduce the solid egg white to a mush (not the original viscous egg white). What seems common to both examples before is that the energy of the window push or the grinder was required only when my design in mind is executed according to my free willed/desired goal (intelligent or not). Left to themselves, both the statue and the solid egg white will never spontaneously become another statue or special gourmet egg white respectively, both will inexorably, with the passage of time and in the absence of any intelligent designer, alter nature's course, and will become dust. This describes a spontaneous exergonic process whose temporal evolution is determined by the particular environmental processes present, because ALL systems observed in nature tend to be minimums of free energy state. Ergo, if we agree as to the self-evident, historically verified evolved order in the structure/function and complexity of social institutions, and if we agree as to the observed/documented order in the evolution of structure/function and complexity in the cosmological domain, and if we agree as to the undeniable structural/functional super-complexity of living species during their ontogenetic/phylogenetic evolution into living systems, then we have to agree, as per preceding honest stipulations, that the order and complexity we witness as time passes, cannot be spontaneous. Instead, they are examples of an endergonic process directed to an unknown end or recurrent cyclic stage(s) beyond our present cognitive capacities to precise/describe or even explain. Ergo, the preceding is consistent with the unexplained physical or metaphysical presence of an intelligent 'designer' whose symbolic/sentential logical representation is up for grabs depending on one's level of intellectual sophistication, genetic, memetic biases, emotions, experiences and other circumstantial variables.

All organic matter found in living systems is the result of endergonic reactions because it required external energy expenditures to fuel their structured conversion and comes from photosynthesis or activated chemistry reactions. The breathing of life into such organic matter is a different story. But that doesn't mean that positive mutational changes and the consequent selective evolution by natural selection are simply 'endergonic', not to mention their being 'blind', or 'random' especially when the 'blind' selection results in a more structured and complex-in-function entity. These negentropic results are not spontaneous in any physico-mathematical system we know of. The self-evident increase in complexity witnessed is always an endergonic process that cannot be always credibly explained as happening at the expense of the immediate environment decrease in energy (exergonic).

We need to escape this vicious cycle/oscillation evolution ←→ intelligent design by either changing our physical laws (thermodynamics) to accommodate metaphysical causality or declaring our human species limitations in ever achieving cognitive certainty. Next best is a probable, best adaptive explanation (model) we can live with and in harmony with our biological, psychic and social needs, whether genetically and/or memetically driven.

Perhaps we should concentrate more on the analysis of the mesoscopic level of existential reality without ever abandoning the informed search for better inferential explanations of relevant objects/events beyond our limited sensory detection/description. Sorry for the 'leit motif'.

As I get wiser and older I no longer feel there is an absolute need to identify noumenal dynamics because it would require an infinite resolution in sense perceptual capacity and an infinite brain capacity to represent and parse all relevant but invisible variables likely to be encountered, i.e., absolute truth is a necessary but unreachable goal for our human species. Inevitably, this unavoidable skepticism forces us to be content with accepting a reality that is consistent with such perceptual and conceptual limitations. Thus one must settle for a dynamic, hybrid existential reality consistent with short-sighted goals of a healthy, solvent and happy life, which ultimately I reduce to a transient moment in time where biological, psychic and social equilibrium is maintained. As you know, by training we feel committed to root our conclusions on good measurements and good mathematical logic to compensate for invisible but relevant factors present. That self-imposed discipline makes us deterministic and teleologically oriented as to causality; that is the reason I have spent 4 book volumes in doing just that. Unfortunately for those in search for ultimate truths, the biological imperative that sustains and protects the living by neuro-humoral mediation will always bias, if not control, our decision-making process no matter how hard we try to be exclusively objective. Reality is always subjective because it finds its meaning inside our hardware/software-limited dynamic physical brain. Emotions play a fundamental role in this life-preserving activity, and is much more than the result of inter-synaptic, neuro-humoral receptor activity. Neuro-humoral activity at receptor sites is only the ontological aspect of the existential reality hybrid.

To illustrate, in the Florida recent murder case trial against Casey Anthony, the media frenzy and the public outrage on the verdict is predicated on their ignorance that all it means is that Casey's guilt could not be established factually, even though she may have in fact committed the crime. This very distinction ontological/factual and epistemo-logical/inferential reality is what separates the physical reductionist and the existential realist that must go on for what is reasonably probable and not politically viable.

I chose to do an experiment with myself while listening to both closing arguments. Already on the first week of testimony I had an intuitive feeling, based on clues from Casey's body language expressions, that she couldn't have formed the conscious, intentional 'mens rea' to kill her biological child. That was confirmed based on evidence presented and verdict. But, the prosecution arguments were also credible at closing arguments and I felt stupid—as a licensed lawyer—in realizing that moment's conclusion that both opposing narratives were probably true! But then I recuperated when I also realized this was not about absolute truth and certainty but about probable truth, all things considered. We pitiful humans . . . .

CHAPTER 13

It is impossible not to feel frustrated about how much time I have spent looking for human answers to unanswerable questions. I have almost completed a lifetime cycle of search for answers to the question of existence, life and conscious free will; that slow, hesitant but unrelenting trip to experience noumenal truth only to end where I started with nothing much to share to advance the cause of humanity. But evolutionary advances, albeit very slow, have definitely been historically recorded. Suzi looks at me with pitiful eyes as if saying "the more things change, the more they remain the same." It is my retirement hobby to follow the drum beats of an internal voice guiding my search . . . "For what?", Ms. Suzi 'Sancho Panza' replies to a saddened Don Quixote that continues his relentless battle with the windmills (human species limitations) thinking they are the super complexities of existence that need solution. We will probably never know for sure but it's fun to at least guess the probability of an occurrence based on our reasoned speculations and conjectures. "Yes, but how have all those predictions improved on the basic animal behavior of the human species,?" Suzi argues, "human relations are even worse even here in the U.S.A." No doubt she has a good point. Should we all become Sartrean existentialists and live from crisis to crisis? We cannot even trust our own introspective self searches for reliable data on which to base our decisions. Are we all 'aka dummies' looking at ourselves in the mirror and believing the reflection we 'see'? Is absolute, introspective self knowledge an illusion? Suzi knew that for the next hours I would be lost in reflective activity and she would lose my company again.

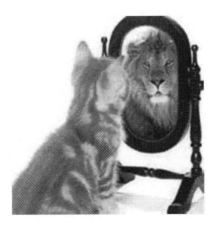

The Spanish philosopher Ortega y Gasset's dictum that humans cannot ever divorce themselves from their ongoing biopsychosocial (BPS) circumstance ("El hombre es el y su circumstancia.") posits for me one of the most intriguing questions about human behavior when confronted with real-time, relevant existential, ongoing contingencies during the decision-making process. Which aspect controls the resulting decision? Can the self always rely on knowing the absolute truth value? If our human species proudly claim being the protagonists of a neo-Copernican revolution that situates us at the very center of the universe because of being uniquely endowed with the marvel of being able to report on a conscious, introspective journey into ourselves, then it is proper to investigate the expected invariance of that solid knowledge base supporting our decision-making activity when confronting and solving contingencies threatening our lives or biopsychosocial equilibrium. The successful evolution of the species depends on the solidity of our self knowledge base so we do not evolve, like other species, as mere creatures of changing circumstances. How is a real-time human being going to find that quotidian solution that is both simultaneously relevant, adaptive and at the same time, transcending its immediate immanent character to become the absolute standard of righteousness independent of any variations in the circumstantial aspects surrounding the specific individualized contingency? From the perspective of a universal standard, can our human species escape his circumstantial shadow that inexorably follows him regardless of his conscious awareness of its possibly negative impact presence? If we were to trust recorded history accounts, only a few individuals successfully resisted the convenience drive of his biopsychosocial circumstance and opted, 'contra natura', to swim against the strong current and altruistically act against self-interest conveniences to set universal standards of behavior for others to emulate in the Ten Commandments Decalon, Tables of the Law, Koran, etc. We call them the historical prophets. What guided them? Where is their source of inspiration and guidance? How is righteousness transformed into a living reality? Informed speculations and conjectures are thus in order to at least answer the how, e.g., the highly speculative BPS sub-model of Reciprocal Transcendental Information Transfer between the human neo cortex and transfinity. At this time, I find it necessary to further expand briefly on the nature of the complex question being asked. Why are some humans in history 'more special" than others connecting with that mysterious 'source' regardless of their preceding formal training in ethics, axiology, etc?

In the following explanation, I will try an objective analytical perambulatory dissection of this issue on how we gain and use knowledge. One can gain ontological knowledge about the immediate external world and internal body-proper phenomenal environment with the aid of instrumental recordings from external receptors as in vision, audition, taste, touch, temperature, etc. or with internal proprioceptors, stretch receptors, muscle spindles, chemoreceptors, etc. We establish their ontological status by the more reliable direct measurements of their structure/function or the less reliable spoken accounts/ reports or explanations of the subjective qualia experienced. Phenomenologically, these real time, ongoing descriptions entail a minimal form of **self**-conscious activity for the experiencing subject due to the immediacy of the object or event being witnessed or otherwise experienced. But, even when we are asked, immediately after the occurrence, to give an account of what happened, how do we know that one's ongoing, particular mental state, beliefs, desires, sensations, etc. did not significantly influence our reply? That particular mental state is very important. It happens to be our persisting **self**, our personality, our identity as quoted by the classical Greeks as 'Gnoscete Ipsum' or 'know thyself.' But, is an 'objective' ontological description being modified by 'subjective' epistemological explanations controlled by our immediate and ongoing mind state or a persisting mental state? What controls the decision-making process, convenient short term expediency or long term ethical and moral universal considerations? Is our '**self-knowledge**' data base persistent or subject to expedient and convenient modifications? Phrased differently, is the decision-making process controlled by an introspective, **conscious** self knowledge or by the **subconscious** genetic and memetic reflex networks? It is the role of the subconscious neuro-humoral control network to provide the necessary adjustments responsible for the biopsychosocial (BPS) equilibrium servo controls, those that make possible for human beings to reflexly respond to familiar situations as recorded in their memory data base. New unfamiliar situations mobilize additional self conscious resources that make it possible to adapt to the potentially dangerous novelty on the basis of either BPS needs or conveniences, immanent or transcendental aspirations and rarely, altruistic acts against self interests. There is a very important distinction to be made between knowledge acquired through perceptual familiarity and knowledge acquired by conceptual representations, i.e., knowledge we *describe* with some certainty and knowledge we *explain* by way of inferential symbolic or sentential logical representations of both physical and non-physical properties. When we make normative logical decisions about the relevant non-physical, extra sensory invisibilities, it is only when they are rooted on the falsifiable, measurable and probable facts about objects and/or events that we can claim to be speaking with a Kantian wisdom, a sort of epistemological naturalism or epistemontology. A reading of Kant's Critique of Pure Reason will explain it better. When the human experience to be communicated resist statistical apprehension by Bayesian logic, we are now in a very different but equally important psychosocial theological manifold which humans individually adopt as our living truths in harmony with their evolving individualized, real time existential circumstance. As we can see, there are many layers in the content of that self knowledge reservoir we tap when making conscious, freely willed decisions. We hope the reader differentiates this time honored, historically recorded, self evident truths from the typical Sartrean existentialism where individuals live and blindly evolve from moment to moment with no normative guidelines to show the righteous way to behave to preserve the viability of the human species. However, the self evident truth is that we, as a species, have evolved in obvious defiance to the also self evident and reliable natural thermodynamic laws of entropy. Why?

Why do some people lead lives exemplifying moral virtues, prudence and courage, benevolence and compassion notwithstanding the many and various temptations to look exclusively after their own ego centered self interests often at the expense of innocent others, like so many currently elected or appointed politicians? Egoism comes in different flavors—psychic, rational or a deadly combination of both when it evolves into a normative rational mindset where the ultimate aim is to unrelently maximize one's **self**-interest at any cost. A veritable intentional psychopathological state of the likes of Hitler, Stalin, Franco, Napoleon and other brilliant historical non-repentant personalities; these are the diametrical opposites of our historical prophets. If these diametrically opposite extremes of historical behavior are conditioned by natural inherited intelligence and not the result of a corresponding circumstantial existential reality, what then is the fundamental difference? In the classical 'Summa Contra Gentiles' it is suggested that through 'divine assistance' some chosen individuals are blessed with a direct and immediate grasp of first principles. This reminds us again to ponder on the nature of that claimed divine assistance as being essentially the ability to harmonize the unavoidable, immanent self BPS interests with the transcendental and universal requirements of virtuosity; like Leibniz conceptualization of theology as a human brain centered effort in the 'chosen ones' to create a "science of law". It is almost impossible for us limited human creatures to conceive of an 'assistance', divine or not, as lacking an efficient physical cause, however small in dimensions. Therein lies the mesmerizing attraction of an epistemology rooted primarily on functional reality as experienced, e.g., the Kantian 'synthetic a priori propositions'; also somewhat reminiscent of Locke's faith on what material substances and their powers can do outside our capability of ever measuring their dimensions or functions. But we can always write about the explanatory poetry of a belief or just muse on sheer 'cult' nonsense. Been there, done that. After all, why deny it, human certainty is nothing but an epistemic property of human subjects communicating their beliefs with the assistance of all kinds of convenient metaphysical logic and other axiomatic contraptions, however practically useful they may turn out to be. For those of us addicted with the curiosity for the identification of noumenal reality or first principles, we have no choice but to rely on the self evident truth that drives our belief-forming activities. Unfortunately the best guide we humans have is what appears to us as counter intuitive, e.g., those non-physical epistemological conceptualizations that become entities able to produce forces that affect physical objects or events. Last but not least, the Darwinian evolution abstraction may be the result of indirect interpretations about observations but it sure as hell makes sense to speculate, if not believe, that species do change in appearance due to what seems to be a natural process that 'selects and maintains' in nature. This may be necessary to explain how species change but may not be sufficient to explain ALL BPS changes experienced inside our quotidian 4d real time existential cage. 'Evolutionary epistemology' is in! We have to live with it until a better epistemological poetry explanation comes into being, especially when analyzing the 'replication' pathway of the selected change. Spontaneously self sustained? If so, we may have to change all of our physics laws that have been so successful in predicting the probability of future events because they **do not** predict a **spontaneous** increase in complexity of structure or function as we corroborate as happening in recorded history. Finally, it is very tempting to assume that acquiring and reporting knowledge about the external environment shouldn't be different when doing the same in respect to ourselves because, if we accept the premise that reality is in our brains, why go elsewhere? But we have to keep looking and continue to write poetry.

We can summarize and easily conclude that there is no doubt that most of us humans rely blindly on our introspective memory accounts of our respective lives because they seem infallible and seem to account for at least all of our acquired existential knowledge. The rest of our knowledge is in genetic data bases we cannot change at will. After all, it seems odd that we should feel that what we are thinking about in any given moment is not true! Yet, how can we be certain we are capable of attaining a third person perspective about our self attributions free from higher order inferences adopted from prefab 'theories of mind' or behavioral influences? Even Dr. Dennet agrees but calls it differently. Interestingly, we have analyzed (see articles on intra and interspecies information transfer) how we may be utilizing same brain circuitry, especially mirror neurons, in gaining reliable insights about our own mental states as we do in others' mental states. In this simulation effort we may learn of other's states of mind by using their facial expression cues in a given situation and then projecting oneself empathically into the other's situation, i.e., allowing the observer through a special mode of self-reflection, to experience what one would believe or desire, feel, etc. if we were in that situation ourselves. We had hoped to use similar arguments to explain how the use of similar brain processing circuitry may be activated when receiving information from transfinity sources, if any. We have argued that this 'simulation theory certainty' needs to be qualified and improved on.

When we are asked to report on our personal account of, e.g., an accident we had just witnessed, how many persons may '**consciously**' report relevant objects, events or sensations 'experienced' but **not** strictly present inside our perceptual field or emotional mindset during the occurrence? Was it influenced by the reporter's current and ongoing mindset or was it objective even when it would carry negative consequences to the reporter or to his special others? Why the inconsistency? Is this the result of the inevitable **subconscious** influence from individualized circumstances, e.g., sensations, emotions, appetites, etc. or was it always the result of a **conscious** deliberate intention to benefit from the consequences? Are we really having those thoughts and sensations reported? Are they true? There is no unanimous consensus as to how to evaluate the results of introspective reports, or what weight to accord 'other sources'. Introspection therefore faces an especially complex problem of "standard of calibration." Should we rely on what often seems to be an exalted epistemic claim made on behalf of introspective self consciousness as being true and very distinct from the brain epistemic processing we use in other domains, i.e., on what credible basis can we claim that there is a fundamental difference between self-knowledge and other-knowledge? What is obviously distinct is the leisurely, scholarly, addictive habit of the few retired to indulge in poetry writing about the complexities of self and the many others sharing the same ecological niche, very different from the quotidian existential reality of the surviving, unemployed and stressed 'many others' coexisting with us. Nothing wrong with writing poetry so long as you keep your feet on the solid grounds of real time existence as you look at the stars for guidance and then take the first step 'ad astra per asperas'.

Suzi calmly observes with innate curiosity how I strain to explain what is not even clear to me as I step down from the clouds into the high horses and then get my feet on solid ground where real-time existence continues unfazed, "time to eat honey." And then, back to existential reality . . . .

For example, how can anyone escape the anguish of witnessing how death lurked in my two older sons' lives? Why not hypothetically become their friends instead of a loving father that has not left a stone unmoved trying to prevent the inevitable? I need to keep living . . . so I tried . . . .

CHAPTER **14**

What is the difference between friendship and love?

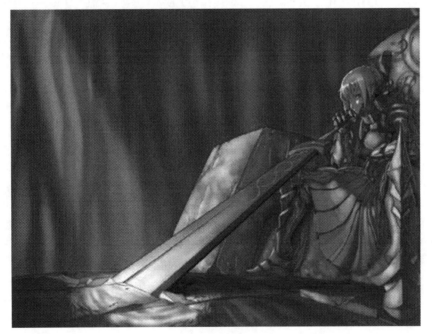

Armor Dark Saber

After having experienced the hurt associated with the loss of her son and husband before she met me, Suzi will understand, I hope, the oddity of my escaping into metaphysical explanations to rationalize my solution to find inner peace and keep going. Bear with me Suzi . . .

The hurtful experience of witnessing the painful journey of my son from a moribund state into the irreversible death and transfiguration, and the concomitant expressions of empathy and love from friends and family everywhere, gave me the opportunity to reflect further on the co-existence of both abstract metaphysical and practical existential aspects of trans-cultural love and friendship as recently identified in the various expressions of condolences from family and friends worldwide, all now briefly analyzed below from a biopsychosocial perspective. Because of the wide trans-cultural spectrum, ranging from my readers whom I have never personally met to biological filiations, I am trying, myself, to understand if friendship and love qualia may be an essential part of the inherited and/or acquired survival instinct or does it transcend the primitive function of keeping the human species together for the common defense against survival threats or against their collective biopsychosocial integrity in order to guarantee the survival and continuation of the species to reproductive age and beyond. Or is it part and parcel of another metaphysical, impersonal, apathetic logical elaboration of the language faculty that expresses a ratification of value and commitment to defend universal values and entities as varied as other species, objects, principles or goals? This metaphysical language processing conceptualize into analytical, abstract, symbolic and sentential representations (metaphors) of the real time existential experience of the grieving actor (whether inherited, acquired and 'revealed') which will stoically and dispassionately bear on his decision-making processes to rationalize the painful quale when accessed. Does it express an abstract but genuine love or an equally genuine existential friendship? Is there a difference? Do we need to choose or do we consciously will, as an adaptive defense mechanism, an ataraxic state to mediate but inevitably execute a compromise between the ontologically, existentially experienced angst and the epistemologically, rationally idealized in abstraction? Before I proceed further in this brief analysis, I need to explain what is the western cultural norm for describing existential love.

Quoting from 1 Cor. 13:4-7, NIV, Apostle Paul described love in the famous poem in 1 Corinthians, thus: "Love is patient, love is kind. It does not envy, it does not boast, it is not proud. It is not rude, it is not self-seeking, it is not easily angered, it keeps no record of wrongs. Love does not delight in evil but rejoices with the truth. It always protects, always trusts, always hopes, and always perseveres." It is self-evident this metaphysical universal-laden quote does **not** describe the behavior of most of us mortal members of the human species. This kind of conscious **impersonal** behavior is drawing heavily from **both** co-existing, neutrally valence-coded brain data bases. One wonders what guides a human being to preferentially transcend his pitiful real time human existence and accordingly learn also to **objectively** love those objects, principles, or goals they value greatly, like Suzi does with all animals and plants. Can one deeply commit oneself to their defense and preservation even when it is possibly threatening their own preservation, e.g., like the historical prophets or the present day conservationists? This is to be distinguished from the essentially **subjective, emotional, consciously interpersonal** bonding outreach of some volunteers with e.g., objects, political or spiritual convictions, animals, etc. This should not be confused with psychopathological cases of paraphilia where sexual delusions become part of the subject's mindset.

We have all experienced the **interpersonal** expressions of love at the ontological level as essentially a biological human effort, not very different from the extinction of hunger or thirst driven by neuro-hormones and characterized by probable sexual attraction and attachment. The latter is better characterized as the psycho-social and cultural acquired component influenced also in its instantiation or embodiment by <u>hormones</u> promoting an experience of mental well being, e.g., <u>oxytocin</u>, vasopressin, <u>neurotrophins</u>, <u>pheromones</u>, etc. The signs and symptoms of this <u>physiological arousal</u> are characterized by transitory, trivial cardio-respiratory dysfunction. An important variation of this interpersonal element is that seen when the epistemological component is in control, i.e., where the experience of affectionate feeling of intimacy and empathy is **not** accompanied by physiological arousal. Is the emotional component totally absent? Quare. When my international friends from HiQ listings and extended distant family that I have not seen or heard from for a long time send cards and e-mails of condolences, do they truthfully say what they mean and mean what they say or is it just a culturally-imposed, emotionally-neutral protocol/language script being followed?

Interestingly, in my mental perambulations in search of tranquility and adequacy of response to suffering, I discovered the <u>Pyrrhonians</u> epistemological approach most convenient because the situation could be handled in theory as an **impersonal** relation. Why assume the love expressions from the stranger are not truly qualia experienced by the sender? I have often discussed with Suzi about the qualia truthfulness of birthday cards scripts. Why not suspend judgment on dogmatic cultural or theological beliefs in the absence of factual evidence or credible intuitions? But more important, one can rationalize the situation and ask the <u>Epicureans</u> question, "Why should I worry about an intention I do not even know exists?" This was the same type of rational liberation from the anguish of the unknown I managed to experience when viewing the dying scenario of my son before my teary eyes, a sort of conscious self-induced tranquil <u>apatheia</u> as long as I have no **rational** way to establish either the physical torment of my dead son or the truth of the intentions of the condolence senders. In retrospect, if I have consistently acted with respect, consideration, praised the trustworthy, being compassionate and affectionate with dissenting colleagues and friends, and consciously have practiced virtuosity (most of the times ☺), why should I worry? If I have consciously behaved that way, I need not be concerned about the valence of love and friendship of others as long as I am able to love and be a good, friendly sentient being. This conscious, tranquil mental state is described by the Greeks as the 'ataraxic' state.

Is this the functional role of the metaphysical, logic-based, universally valued metaphor abstractions that the language faculty codes for our human species to "consciously" access when in need to search for an adaptive BPS tranquil state, however immanent and transient?

In closing, a note to my local and international friends, family and colleagues: Please accept my sincere thanks for your cards, phone calls and e-mails offering your condolences for the untimely death of our beloved sons. Your thoughtfulness will be long remembered. I hope Suzi understands my questioning of commercial scripts to be found in commercial cards. What is important is that it coincides with your true feelings and if not, you become committed to try to live up to the written expressions you adopted, so help you God.

I promise I will have one more account of how I was able to rationalize my painful experiences to save my mental self from inner self destruction because love is a "saber" with two sharp cutting edges.

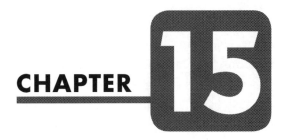

CHAPTER 15

Rationalizing life & existence to escape painful qualia.

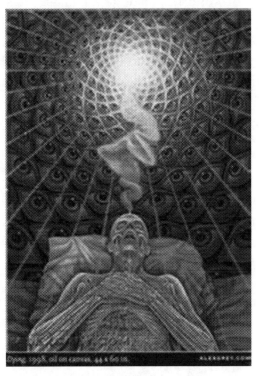

Death and Transfiguration

Once I had survived the ineffable experience of being a living witness of the untimely death and transfiguration of my two loving, older sons, the only way I knew to keep going was to escape suffering and frustration by fantasizing reality as my close friends and family describe it. I know of no other way to escape the pain that started as soon as I was able to distinguish self from others. Bear with me again in this last chapter.

We, as individuals, seem to be controlled by two, often disparate, existential systems, each endowed with its own distinct strategy when processing the idea of life and the circumstance of quotidian, real time existence and death. Both existential mind sets, conscious and subconscious, respectively, can significantly change our behavioral handling of unexpected contingencies such as actually coming face to face with impending death and suffering as was my case. The epistemological/ abstract eternal and the ontological/individualized experiential, clash in both attitudes and actions as the will, many times, works out adaptive solutions in very different—almost opposite—ways. The coexistence of both conscious and subconscious strategies comes dramatically into life when experiencing and/or witnessing the metaphysical and emotional evolution of a human death experience. I have been obsessed about life and consciousness for as long as I have been able to think. Here is a short chronology of how now, at the sunset of my productive life, I have almost completed a full cycle and I repeat, the more essential things change, the more they remain almost the same for us pitiful humans.

Life. At the risk of being repetitious I still remember many years back, when I was a young Catholic biophysicist at Sloan-Kettering Institute for Cancer Research, I was very curious about how a white crystalline ribonucleic acid (RNA) powder (Rous Sarcoma Virus or RSV) standing in a test tube for weeks could come 'alive' when cultured with chick embryo fibroblasts cells in culture. I couldn't wait to capture and describe for my doctoral thesis that crucial moment of life animation by recording serial measurements with the latest biophysical chemistry technology including electron microscopy. Then I was lost and threw in the towel as my RSV disappeared from view inside the cellular cytoplasm. What happened to the electron microscope? The huge electron microscope seemed to 'apologize' to anxious me. Soon afterwards RSV was found by somebody else to have <u>incorporated itself</u> into the fibroblast cell host nuclear DNA. And soon afterwards Howard and Temin won a Nobel Prize by describing how an RNA transcriptase enzyme enabled the viral replication based on similar results. At that time, I simply called the RSV crystal a 'truncated life' who hijacked the host cell's reproductive machinery for its own cancerous replicating ends. I then decided to come back to that 'life enigma', in a neurophilosophical broader context upon retirement.

Today, after four published volumes and a 'Treatise' on a model of brain dynamics, the problem has become more complex than I had bargained for, as will be briefly discussed below.

The main Gordian knot has been an un-necessary quest by physical scientists and metaphysical theologians alike for a monadic interpretation of life at the exclusion of the other. Our contribution has been to argue for what's worth on both sides of the same coin.

Scientific methodology has failed to explain how life, albeit in apparent or presumed abeyance of the first and second law of thermodynamics, is able to **spontaneously** evolve into a complex structural and dynamic entity able to self-generate and sustain a super-complex intrinsic order; all allegedly without the benefit of a preceding blueprint for such specific destiny. The fundamental transition from inorganic/organic atoms and molecules into a living unit of life still remains a fundamental mystery in physics, chemistry, and biology because of a lack of empirically complete and consistent descriptions or explanations of life as an emergent, irreducible and animated fact of nature, including Dr. Dennet's . . . and my own of course for that matter.

One can understand why the comfort of giving some rest to an unsatisfied inquiring mind by resting the case on a convenient "self-replicating" DNA which understandably has evolved into a major metaphor for explaining **all** there is to be learned about life. After all, why not invoke coding self-replicators and coded self-organizing interactors at all levels of organization to evasively counteract the inescapable and self-evident causally efficient but invisible driving force which seems to be controlling evolution by natural selection? However, it is just as counter-intuitive to analytical logic to conceptualize humans as survivalist epiphenomenal gene-vehicles, a la Dawkins or Dennet, as it is to invoke the **exclusive** mediation of an intelligent design force or blueprint guiding such beautiful and complex order defying natural laws as witnessed in developmental and evolutionary biology. What IS life then? Let's first agree on the terminology. What do we mean by 'life', 'existence', 'essential' as opposed to 'accidental' attributions, and other ambiguities.

Having personally witnessed the early death and transfiguration of my dear son John Arthur, I had the opportunity to differentiate between that conceptualized instant of animation of matter when 'life' comes into being, like the RSV ribonucleoprotein described above, and that subsequent, perceptual description of 'life in transit' that I chose to call 'existence' in real time.

Central to 'life' is its **scientific** characterization of 'existence' as essentially open-ended systems **yet** subtly maintained in steady states and **yet** far from an equilibrium, all sustained by a self-regulated inflow/outflow of matter/energy to fuel self-regulated auto-catalytic smaller cycles. The latter are somehow programmed to complete a much larger human life cycle of simultaneously conjoined endergonic negentropy and exergonic entropy. In the beginning of the cycle—the endergonic control phase—we sense and respond to internal and external environments, we extract energy, build and generate complex sub-systems at a faster rate than at a later exergonic control phase where we degrade energy, deconstruct and degenerate at faster rates as we complete our human cycle of life, happiness, suffering and eventual death. Living is dying, but only for the individual. The species continues to evolve. As we learn more and more about the biophysical chemistry of living

organisms, we seem to be in denial that, because we cannot ontologically describe either a causally efficient force to drive the dynamics of the living or the essential negentropy of structural/functional details of its self-evident order, there must exist an epistemological metaphysical entity providing the blueprints for their orderly evolution into a living unit. So, why not ignore those two postulates of scientific methodology and invoke the mysterious existence of autopoietic, self generating, self-sustaining, super-complex activity that, equally mysteriously 'emerges' into a super-complex living unit? As such, that miracle of creation is seen as being somehow essentially endowed with another super-complex genetic and memetic memory database good for a human life cycle, a materialistic act of faith and denial. So much for the super-complexity of the enactment of life from the non-living.

What about the evolutionary path of the living unit as it unfolds in real space-time? Do we evolve according to the exclusively rational ontological model of the materialistic faith or the exclusively epistemological model of the theological faith? What kind of decision-making behavior, should we predict from either model? Are there other alternatives? Stay tuned for a rehash of the same, all explained and crunched into less than a thousand pages, an epistemontological model of conscious reality. See also Harold 2001.

It has not been so bad for an ontological scientific model of 'life' rooted essentially on falsifiable sense-phenomenal measurements on the one hand and intuitions about experiences on invisible and significant objects and/or events whose existential meaning is epistemologically found when expressed and communicated in a metaphysical logic language, on the other hand, a hybrid model of sorts. But which side of the epistemontological coin do we choose? Do we need to have choices?

Existence. Contrary to the experience of the originally elongated chick embryo fibroblast that predictably got transformed into a spherical tumor cell within the standard environmental temperature and pressure condition (STP) of the experiment, in the exclusive case of the human species, existence is an individualized, self-conscious experience of being oneself. This is distinct from the relevant sense-phenomenal or intuited invisible surroundings which become the human existential circumstance. Yet we are inseparably joined together in most cases. The human existence is predicated on inherited, acquired or willfully (or not) created circumstances. The latter does not exclude circumstances from being consciously willed (or not) as imaginary, mythical, fictional, and the like. To say that it 'exists' means/ implies it is 'real' for a self-conscious person within a stated probability. If the object/event is a pathognomonic reality of mental disease it is **not** proper to say it 'exists'. If something 'is', whether ontologically sensed or epistemologically inferred as probable (not possible!) under specified STP conditions, then it 'exists' under the scrutiny of metaphysical logic methods even if invisible to the sensory detection. In other words, existence implies a probable predicate attribution of an entity that 'is', ontologically measured matter or an epistemologically inferred micro mass because of extrasensory dimensions. It is important to distinguish further between the existential—as defined—and the predicative context. There is an essential and an accidental predicate. A particulate matter is an **essential** predicate— invisible or not to human detection—whereas a wave form is an **accidental** predicate expressing the manner in which the particulate matter travels in space time. Color, shape, etc. are examples of accidental, non-essential predicates. Of more common use are, unfortunately, **identity** predicates where equivalent essential or

accidental features are substituted for the original and then the **representation** handled as if they 'existed' in reality and not analogically, a serious categorical error often found in the literature. Thus man is **essentially** a genetically determined biological entity with environmentally determined, acquired **accidental** predicates such as temperament, color, stature, and other psychosocial attributions. It should be obvious that once there exist accidental predicates there has to be an implied essential predicate because the former cannot have an independent existence. "Man" is he and his circumstance, a truly biopsychosocial (BPS) hybrid with free will. Without an introspective self consciousness-based free will, one can conceive of a BPS adapted sub-human living being whose behavior or decision making process can be explained by Skinnerian operant conditioning or simulated in a computer. It is both the introspective capacity and the consequent co-generation of a silent proto language and thought that is exclusively human, as argued elsewhere. Having outlined the primacy of the genetically driven **biological** imperative of self preservation under unconscious control as an **essential** predicate and the memetically driven **accidental** predicate of his **psycho-social** existential circumstances under subconscious control, we should be in a position to generalize a model predicting the decision-making process for the human species. Which aspect will carry more weight in the free willing of behavioral adaptive alternatives, the rational or the emotional? Both, in most cases. The human species has been able to transcend the coded alternatives programmed in his genetic and memetic data bases and improvise a very individualized adaptive response tailored to his ongoing existential circumstance at that particular instance, sometimes contrary to his own BPS interests. When you objectively ponder on this scenario, you will realize that the materialistic, physicalist approach rooted exclusively on scientific methodology, while necessary and persuasive, is not sufficient to adequately model the dynamics of life and existence. We need to complement the physical evolutionary approach with a metaphysical component that will reach outside our 4-d space time for answers as explored in one of our dissertations. Of course, one can always settle for a myopic invocation of the magic of multiple auto-poetic, self generated and self sustained forces that magically and spontaneously 'emerge' into a super complexity that violates the very physico-mathematical foundations of the physicalist rational approach. What role do non-rational, emotional circumstances play in the survival of our human species? What follows was my deliberate, non-classic way of dealing with powerful emotions that threatened to control my life, like a family death can.

Death and Transfiguration. As my teary eyes watched my son Johnny die I kept asking myself when does life end? Does life refer more to the functional integrity of the metabolic machinery sustaining the vital homeostatic processes like cell respiration and generation or does it mean the sudden or gradual extinction of that integrated 'animation' of matter we normally describe as being 'alive'? For most of us parents, it is more like experiencing an irreversible harrowing process where both aspects exist, the biological chronicle of 'systems failure' and the sudden extinction of all measurable indices of animation. The former is **described** by the physical credo that models the scientific physicalist script, the latter is **explained** by the metaphysical script that models the theological credo. This inextricable duality makes life and death impossible to disambiguate. Having accepted death as a permanent, irreversible event, it now looks like the virtual mirror image of birth **and** life is seen now as 'something' that moves in and out of matter. But we may synthesize complex matter in the laboratory but never living/animated matter as described above. The combination of both sex gametes' DNA at fertilization to 'synthesize' living matter has always required a living cellular environment. Perhaps we will never know how 'life' was carried or induced at conception.

As I pondered and grieved, I turned my focus on the comparative effects of this ongoing process of the dying, and myself on two levels. The first level was an evaluation of the efficacy of interspecies information transfer between Johnny and me. The second level was a speculation as to his suffering vis-a-vis my own. It did not take long for me to realize that the un-natural analgesic and anxiolytic pharmacological effects on both observed and observer respectively would seriously interfere with our cortical pre-motor mirror neurons and limbic systems as amply discussed elsewhere in one of my books. When he was still in denial of the seriousness of his condition, his facial musculature profile and mental alertness reflected his hopes for recovery. When he was close to death his facial musculature relaxed as his mindscape revealed confusion and/or acceptance of his condition; at one point he even smiled as I broke down in tears. Not being able to analyze much at the first level, I turned into a speculation as to whether towards the end he was still suffering at least as much as I did. I was surprised at what a self-induced rationalization of the ongoing experience can do. At that point, it became much clearer the distinction between the unconscious, subconscious and introspective self-consciousness aided by the co-generation of silent language and thought. I re-discovered, as hinted in a previous publication, that ultimately, rationalization of existential reality is a self-serving activity geared to provide an experience of biopsychosocial well being, an epicurean hedonistic goal!! Following are the tentative arguments I fashioned in my head inside the Hospice room on that Sunday before Johnny finally died. Nobody wants their lives to end unless in agonizing pain, not the case of Johnny. But 'it' can move in at birth and out of existence at death, i.e. if there is re-incarnation, life is like an intervening gap of non-instantiated hibernation, and death is a sort of break from 'existence' in the real, dangerous world and will continue in a paradisiac sleep state waiting for a subsequent second or third coming . . . Epicurus is smiling in his animated hibernation!

Epicurus characterized death as a harrowing evil but then rationalized: "to whom?" Not to Johnny. Death will not affect him because when alive it is absent and when it comes, he is absent. For death to harm the subject who dies, there must exist a *subject* who is harmed by death to satisfy its causal efficiency. Furthermore, who can precise the nature of the *harm* and the *time and place* where that harm is materialized? Restating, when the subject is alive there is no death and after we die there is no living subject to be harmed. Ergo, grief is entirely self-centered. I, the father, who wrapped myself inside a blanket of self-pity and guilt, emotionally grieve at my possible indirect, un-intentional involvement in his demise. But Johnny's body and mind are not harmed by its own extinction. If we ponder hard and find out we did everything a parent can do to preserve his life, we can be harmed **only** by whatever real negative deeds that will cause us or others to suffer. Is this the unavoidable, self serving or self-preserving BPS integrity function of self consciousness, to rationalize an escape hatch and survive as a species? We have examined in detail how humans can logically analyze a situation in abstract, with the best of our analytical faculties during a decision-making contingency, only to find out how the individualized, ongoing, real time existential reality hijacks the logical justifications in providing the subject with a feeling of biopsychosocial equilibrium and a sense of well being. Needless to say, this behavior may be illegal, immoral and, in the long run, may even constitute an act against self interest. But this is not always the case where altruistic acts against self-preservation interests are in conscious control of the decision-making brain circuitry. There have been recently published fMRI studies on decision-making choices of alternatives demonstrating the individualized nature of these processes where ongoing, real-time experiences seem to counter well thought analytical conclusions in the subjects tested. If the experience and peremptory satisfaction of a sense of biopsychosocial well being controls our existential reality, then what can we say about the prophets that, living under similar or worse existential circumstances before the influence of organized religions, were able to overcome those strong neuro-humoral emotional satisfaction drives and do the right thing where self interest was not in exclusive control of behavior? What guided their sacrificial behavior against self-interest? There is definitely more to come on this issue.

The living human species, and to a large extent other subhuman species, share a wide spectrum of properties and phenomena that are entirely absent from inanimate matter. Living organisms undergo metabolic activity, grow and differentiate, respond to sensory stimulation, move, develop complex, organized functional structures, show the results of inherited environmental fluctuations, reproduce, and die. They also develop significant ecological adaptive fitness to changing environments. This is the kind of behavior that a complex program can make a robot to perform without the choice of deciding not to comply as a conscious will. Can the rationalized metaphor of the epistemological human abstraction be separated from the circumstantial, ontological human of our historical experience? Quare. This is precisely what we find in controlled and falsifiable studies.

The physical aspects of biological lives involves not only the replication of the nucleic acids that carry the genetic information, the memetic/epigenetic growth and maturation of the organism through a sequence of developmental steps that, exclusively in the case of humans, includes the ability to introspectively discover his individualized identity as distinct from others' and the surroundings. The discovery of self co-evolves with the faculty of a language faculty now able to represent existential reality as metaphors which most likely share an embodiment with other vital neuronal networks in the brain real estate. Like other animals, inherited and environmentally-acquired servo controls guide the genetic and epigenetic preservation of biological life and its relevant neuro-humoral concomittants.

Unlike other animals, humans, in addition, rely on their unique ability of being conscious of self and others and evolve the language faculty for communication with self and others in creating a safe and progressive social environment fit for reproductive and creative social conviviality. Is the mind's conscious linguistic representation of existential reality as conceptual metaphor abstractions separate from the quotidian unconscious/subconscious servo control of behavior? Can the physical sense-phenomenal, perceptual data bases and their metaphysical metaphor representations thereof both instantiated/embodied and share common neuronal networks? If so, which one is in control in the decision-making process? Quare . . . it all depends. If we depend on recorded history, we would have to conclude that by and large experiencing the satisfaction of an adapted biopsychosocial equilibrated well being at the very moment when a decision must be made will trump any other logically-based abstraction or altruistic motive. Only by exception will anyone negate the exemplary lives of historical prophets to be guided by the larger, transcendental view of the metaphor abstraction coded by the language faculty; many times performing conscious altruistic acts contrary to self interests. Why so? Are they aliens from another galaxy, immune from the pains and tribulations of existential reality or are they privy to extrasensory guidance information, e.g., revelations?

Lakoff, in his seminal work on 'Embodied cognition' 1963, in open defiance of Chomskian language dogma that grammar was independent of meaning, had already considered the idea that the mind is not only represented in the brain, but that the physical brain is causally efficient in controlling the metaphysical mind and not the other way around! Except in the cases of the historical prophets. However counter-intuitive as it may sound, it is a self-evident fact of life for the majority of us mortals. To our knowledge, nobody has even tried to understand the details of this neuronal network instantiation /embodiment of language representations as universals, as metaphor or virtual reflections on existential reality. Thus, to understand the meaning of life and consciousness (not robotic awareness) we must cross disciplines, both the ontological perceptual of the natural physical sciences and the epistemological conceptual of metaphysical logic and adopt a hybrid epistemontological approach because our cognition of life and existence, that precedes every decision-making act, is influenced, if not determined, by our individualized experiences in the real time physical world. In my opinion there may have been a basic grammar structure, a la Chomsky, that enable communication to satisfy early basic childhood needs and then became the subject of a continuous evolution guided by psycho-social adaptive strategies, a type of generative semantics where much of our language structure derives from physical environmental interactions during the first few years of life. Lakoff and Johnson's '**Metaphors We Live By'** can explain it better. What else can one say about existence?

In case you did not notice, which I doubt, this is an embellished account of my experiences, as I would like people to remember me and not necessarily as they were, especially if it would reveal unintentional bad behavior as driven by circumstances not entirely within my control. We are not perfect and largely a creature of circumstances largely outside our abilities to effectively influence. But those circumstances we can still impact and change in a positive way. We have the moral obligation to become the agents of change according to our capacities to do so. If you are able to and consciously would not, then you are living at the level of subhuman species, not better than your nice dog. If you enjoy that robotic enslavement, so be it and God bless you just the same.

CHAPTER 16

I think that sacrifice is inherent to love and care for others than self. Both Suzi and I loved our pets and each other, and the existential sacrifices all concerned were willing to make in the conclusion of our marital relationship was not necessarily inconsistent with their nobility and Christian values. I was grieving and hurting badly.

While planning to pick up my daughters coming for a weekend visit I confess to my estranged wife Suzi that I still loved her and want her to reconsider her plans of moving back home to Virginia. It is abundantly clear that in Suzi's mind, I had abandoned her for another escape into intellectual dreaming, the result of being overwhelmed by our many family issues. Suzi suggests that her remorse is due to my escapes into conceptual reality where nobody is hurt. She is sacrificial and has no time and space to think, the die is cast. This rift has caused major problems and has triggered the typical insecurity angst and rebellion qualia of the 60's generation amongst my 3 surviving daughters and son in dire need for valuable time to resolve their own health and potential unemployment worries. But Suzi was determined to give in into what she thought was her destiny, with total un-intended disregard for everything that was left behind, a broken home, pets and teary me.

Once again, I relied on my careful handling of our past relationship after my first wife died and was able to feel there was nothing I could do to reverse the recent events. I also deliberately got distracted away with my perambulations in search for an understanding of life and consciousness, the same search I had now extended to include me and the behavior that may have caused this rift. I decided then to take my visiting daughters back to Maryland. So we drove north and stopped at Virginia asking my daughters to continue home that I would join after a brief sojourn, again searching for answers for that mysterious self annihilating behavior of Suzi, curiosity and love are a disease. So, they dropped me at the outer banks at a friendly bed-and-breakfast joint for the weekend while she's hopefully resting at her lifetime friend Carol's home, a few miles away. The motel I was staying was your typical rustic, romantic abode, right on the beach, where the North Atlantic wavelets traveled to the surf at high tide.

I was one of many guests for that long holiday weekend. There was me, pitiful Yogi, a very antisocial, un-engaging TYPE A personality neuroscientist arriving at the inn with my own charged emotional baggage. I couldn't hold back the unending trail of flashbacks about my dear Labrador-chow Charlie Boy and the Memaw cats, I was sure Miss Kitty, the feral cat, was already dead trying to find her way back to her native Deltona, Florida. God knows, I may one day greet her back at the shores of Lake Louise in Deltona. Above all I kept thinking about Suzi sitting near the table surrounded by her breathing equipment struggling to breathe, looking for a pack of menthol lights cigarettes within her addictive sight. I couldn't hold back my tears in front of the bar tender who lifted his eyes momentarily as he poured some Michelob dark beer inside my tall 12 ounce glass while I avoided direct eye contact by swinging my tall chair towards the stormy ocean landscape. I was beginning to wonder how I could possibly call her on the phone. I had no car and the weather was turning ugly, a storm was moving in. But I was on a mission. I picked up my unpredictable cell phone and nervously dialed her number, hoping she still owned the same one she had when she disappeared forever from my life. I got a response, as if she had been waiting for my call. My heart was beating fast and I walked outside so I could hear better. The wind was beginning to sing like Charlie-Boy's howling dog sounds. After a brief exchange of pleasantries, I told her where I was staying and without thinking, typical Suzi, she said "wait for me, I'll be there soon in a blue car, I'll honk twice when I arrive." Before I could reply she hung up saying "I love you". That was my Suzi alright.

There she is now arriving in a blue Chevy. You could always trust her determination. I was awakened from my brief mental trip by virtual Chevy, the black cat that stayed in Deltona, still helplessly looking for his Suzi, and by two loud honks from the car. I ran to the car to open her door, like in the good old times, I could not contain my tears again! What a curse to erupt my inner feelings like a volcano without a control. I didn't care, she was used to this embarrassing spectacle. I hugged her, put my arm around her shoulder and walked her back into the motel. I could feel with my finger the cloth texture of a familiar dress. Of course, it was the unforgettable white linen dress I was attracted to when I first met her at Hospice when grieving for our respective dead spouses. We walked in to a table overlooking the graying Atlantic Ocean as she would have expected and probably predicted for a Piscean like me.

We dined together, sipped red Cabernet Sauvignon as I watched every muscle of expression on her face as she knew I would be doing, trying to read what's in her subconscious mind before she told me. She was beautiful to my biased eyes and nervous as usual. Several naturally aging white hairs were cascading down to her darkened eyebrows covering the also natural signs of frontal fissures. We shared trivial recent short stories before eventually turning nervously to each other as if pleading for emotional comfort. Almost as if a genuine first sight romance had been reborn.

I opened up, at every moment praying that my calm, slow and good mannered views on things would not be misconstrued as if preaching and criticizing. This was her standard misconception of viewing me, the typical retired professor, ex-catedra—as always riding up in a tall high horse, ready to pass judgments on her nervous demeanor and experiences. Far from it.

As always, I always felt guilt and regretted passing up a typical fatherly relationship with my beautiful family of 3 sons and 2 daughters in favor of a busy professional career as a university professor, a practicing medical malpractice lawyer and now—upon retirement—as a make believe neurophilosopher workaholic in training.

I tried real hard to project into Suzi my premonition of seeing her struggling, for what likely will be unbearable days of grief and suffering dictated by her chronic obstructive respiratory condition and her negative family experiences. She looked to me in sadness as she nervously clenched her ever-present pack of menthol light cigarettes. At the same time, I was trying very hard to convince her of somehow slowly approaching her direct family until the eventually wiser and more mature others provide a turning point in their relationship allowing her to begin to deal with her anticipated via crucis. She can always become the protagonist of that wisdom she is capable of and teach them by example her own special living story of a very special type of love and encouraging them to seek that out for themselves in a not so distant future, someday when she will become history. But she was not really listening to me and I was not sure this attention deficit was intentional. Anyway it was time for me to stop preaching and start listening to her familiar side of the story.

After realizing she was not really telling me anything I had not heard robotically repeated, I waited patiently and then suggested a walk outside. I was not making my point across what nature and circumstances imposed as a barrier. Why God?, I asked in silence.

Taking, hand in hand, that quiet sojourn along the grayish and humid beach seascape was a respite from Suzi's heart-rending subconscious script. How sad, I complained to my God; why do you do that to her . . . . and to me? She projected a long look that could have reached outer space in search of something unknown. I also searched in vain for any sign of Antares, looking in vain for the constellation Scorpio where my mother, my uncle and my two older sons patiently await for me with open arms.

Suddenly we were both synchronized on the famous painting of the beach dancers on top of our chimney back in Florida. She held my hand and we danced on the beach sand as I held her tight to my chest when she cried and walked to the blue car. I followed her and opened the car door for her. She was teary and hesitant and Suzi was finally able to kiss me goodbye. I watched the car speed away into the paved road heading back to what I prayed would be her final abode of health, happiness and social acceptance. Goodbye Love . . . .

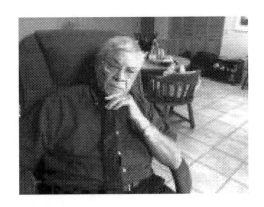

Web Site: http://delaSierra-Sheffer.net

Recent publications:
http://www.lulu.com/browse/search.php?fListingClass=0&fSearch=Dr.+Angell+O.+de+la+Sierra

My Blogs:
https://angelldls.wordpress.com/
http://pulse.yahoo.com/_VHN6HSYWK3LTKWCTZZFCKR2C3U/blog